"Dr. Nair makes a compe  the root cause for cancer and othe solid scientific support for its prevention with anti-inflammatory therapies. An excellent resource for both the public and the medical profession."

Erika Schwartz, MD
Wellness and Prevention Author, *The Hormone Solution*
www.drerika.com

"Our health and that of our loved ones is important. Treat Dr. Nair's book as an educational tool which will enable us to better understand, assess, and choose the best course of treatment when a health problem arises, and how to prevent health problems such as cancer from developing in the first place. It could save our life."

Howard Peiper, ND, nominated for a Pulitzer Prize, has written several best-selling books on nutrition and natural health.
www.walkthetalkproductions.com

"This is an excellent book which is clearly written and easy to read for both lay persons and those working in the field of Health Care. The information presented in Dr. Nair's book provides a comprehensive description of the role of nutrition and the importance of phytochemicals in combination with daily regimes including meditation and exercise, as powerful weapons in helping win the battle against disease. I would heartily recommend this book to all those interested in trying to improve/maintain their health or the health of others."

Margaret R. Ritchie, Ph.D,
Honorary Research Fellow, Napier University, Edinburgh, Scotland;
Former Research Fellow, Bute Medical School, University of St. Andrews, Scotland; Member, Royal Society of Chemistry & Fellow of the U.K. Royal Society of Medicine; Co-Author of *Complementary and Alternative Medicine, a text for health-care professionals*

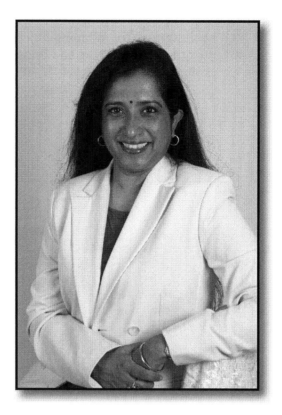

About the Author

Dr. Vijaya Nair is an esteemed researcher and epidemiologist. A native of Singapore, she earned her medical degree from the National University of Singapore. Dr. Nair later immigrated to the United States, where she received a master's degree in epidemiology from Columbia University and completed her post-doctoral fellowship at Harvard Medical School. Fascinated by her studies, Dr. Nair went on to serve as a Professor of Epidemiology at Columbia University, Mailman School of Public Health in New York City. An internationally renowned speaker, Dr. Nair has authored numerous research publications in her quest to educate the public about the health benefits of nature's most powerful anti-inflammatory remedies. In recognition of her expertise, she was invited to submit a paper and deliver an address at the most recent International Translational Cancer Conference. She currently serves as President and CEO of Essence of Life, LLC, a New York based manufacturer of the JIVA Essence of Life line of products. She may be contacted through the Essence of Life website: www.jivasupplements.org.

PREVENT CANCER
Strokes, Heart Attacks and other Deadly Killers!

Dr. Vijaya Nair Reveals Evidence-based
Anti-Inflammatory Healing Remedies

Dr. Vijaya Nair

Cover and book design by Joanna Lee Davis

ISBN 1-884820-92-1
ISBN 13: 978-1-884820922
Library of Congress Catalog Card Number 2008938667
1. natural health 2. cancer 3. inflammation 4. alternative medicine
Printed in the United States of America

Published by Safe Goods Publishing
561 Shunpike Rd., Sheffield MA 01257
www.safegoodspub.com
888-628-8731

Introduction
How I came to write this book

"Happiness lies, first of all, in health."
-George William Curtis (American writer, 1824-1892)

If you're like me, you're keenly interested in preserving or regaining your health, yet you reserve a healthy dose of skepticism about anything promoted as a "miracle cure." I'll be the first to acknowledge that many of the natural supplements available today have big claims but little scientific backing. Too often, when you dig a little deeper you'll find these claims are either distortions of the truth or downright fabrications. So for much of my life I, like many people, disregarded herbal therapies as a valid possibility for the prevention and treatment of serious diseases such as cancer, cardiovascular disease, and Alzheimer's.

When you look at my background you may understand why. Although I was born in Singapore, an island nation in Southeast Asia, my academic studies were similar to that of any Western doctor. I was initially trained as a psychiatrist (a medical doctor who specializes in mental health) in my home country. I later moved to the United States and completed my post-doctoral fellowship at Harvard Medical School and at Columbia University. I then taught epidemiology (the study of identifying risk factors for disease) at Columbia. If I was going to be convinced of the validity of herbal therapies I had to see factual evidence!

However, my unquestioning support of Western medicine started to crack while I was doing research at Columbia. In all the studies I was coming across and helping to direct, one thing was striking — conventional treatments for chronic illnesses had shocking and often painful side effects. For example, standard cancer treatments such as chemotherapy and radiation not only made people sick to their stomachs, bone-achingly tired, and skinny as a rail, but sometimes the side effects were so severe they actually killed the patient! Sadly, many patients were not even told what the risks of these drugs were or how they were going to affect them before starting treatment.

Worse yet, these treatments weren't even helping us win the war against cancer. Despite $200 billion dollars invested in conventional cancer treatments since 1970, as of 2002, Western medicine hadn't made a dent in the rate of cancer deaths.[1] In fact, the U.S. death rate from cancer remained unchanged from 1950 to 2002.[2] So what we had were highly toxic treatments that were not actually saving people's lives. I started to wonder if there was a better way.

Cancer Incidence
By Clifton Leaf March 22, 2004 (Fortune Magazine)

- $200 billion spent since 1970
- 1.56 million papers
- 150,855 experimental studies published on mice
- 10.9 million cases per year (1.5M in USA)
- 6.7 million people die every year (563,700 in USA)

I didn't have to wait long to get my answer. While at Columbia I came upon some promising research on a botanical therapy called cultured soy, showing it held great promise for people with terminal cancers and chronic infections (You'll read more about cultured soy in *Chapter Three*). I read through all of the studies with great interest. Then, I interviewed some of the scientists who conducted the research to find out more about their methodologies and results. Subsequently I had a whole team at Columbia — general practitioners, oncologists (doctors who specialize in cancer), and biostatisticians (people who apply statistics to biology) — review the data. We were convinced the therapy had potential.

That's when I started to get excited. If there was something safe and natural that could improve the quality of life for people undergoing very challenging conventional medicines for very difficult chronic illnesses, then it needed to be investigated seriously. Something inside me knew this was my calling.

For six years I collaborated with various research centers across the globe and worked one on one with cancer patients to study the effects of cultured soy. The results were nothing short of amazing. In fact, the case reports I compiled won recognition from the Office of Cancer Complementary and Alternative Medicine (OCCAM) at the National Cancer Institute. As this book goes to press, a human clinical study is being conducted at The University of Texas M.D. Anderson Cancer Center on using cultured soy to treat the complications of cancer.

While I was busy studying cultured soy, another researcher, Dr. Bharat B. Aggarwal, was doing groundbreaking work with curcumin, a constituent of the herb turmeric. Dr. Aggarwal was arriving at similar conclusions about curcumin's ability to fight chronic disease that the Columbia team had realized about cultured soy. Of course, we weren't the only ones studying botanical therapies for disease prevention and treatment. Other researchers were publishing equally exciting studies on herbal ingredients such as resveratrol, ginger, lutein, ashwaghanda, and green tea. What I learned through reviewing all the research being published was that successful botanical therapies for preventing and treating chronic diseases have one thing in common: they all fight inflammation. Inflammation is your immune system's way of protecting you from physical trauma or foreign invaders, such as viruses and bacteria. It's supposed to be a short and powerful response. But sometimes the body doesn't turn off the inflammation switch and it ends up destroying the very tissues and organs it was meant to protect. We tend to think of inflammation as synonymous with arthritis. However, inflammation can strike anywhere in your body. It's a major contributor to heart disease, cancer, Alzheimer's, and many more life-threatening conditions. Control inflammation and you control disease.

Pouring over those scientific studies, I had an "aha!" moment. I realized this information was too valuable to sit in complicated medical journals, unread by the lay reader. It was at that moment that I decided to devote my life to educating people about nature's most powerful anti-inflammatory remedies.

A few years later, I got to experience the healing power of natural remedies first-hand. In 2004, I started experiencing heavy bleeding. The bleeding was so severe that I had to have a blood transfusion. It turned out I had uterine fibroids — a benign type of tumor that grows in the wall of the uterus. The doctors recommended I get a hysterectomy, which involves the removal of the uterus. But I resisted. I was working with cultured soy at the time and decided to see if taking it, along with some other herbs, would help me. Remarkably, the bleeding stopped and my energy was restored.

For almost a year, I was well. Then the bleeding returned. Again, it was recommended that I get a hysterectomy. Again, I decided against surgery, but this time I realized my body was trying to tell me something; I wasn't taking care of myself. At the time I had a very rigorous schedule. I was working as a researcher. I was traveling back and forth to Asia frequently. I was leading seminars in New York City to hundreds of people every week. And I was going through a divorce. It was too much. I had to stop everything and rest. This time, instead of just taking a few herbs I created an entire wellness program for myself.

First, I underwent a very minor, non-invasive radiological technique to cauterize my uterine arteries instead of the major surgery that was being recommended. Then, based on the fact that my uterus was severely inflamed, I began taking both cultured soy and curcumin together. I also started meditating, got massages and went to therapy to see what in my life was no longer working. Soon, the fibroids began to shrink. In fact, after awhile they shrank 70 percent. Today, my uterus is healthy again.

I know from personal experience that it is possible to create natural, vibrant health using the techniques laid out in this book. If after reading it, just one person finds relief from their suffering or learns how to prevent some of the most debilitating diseases we face today, then I will consider myself successful.

May you enjoy a long and healthy life, free of suffering and disease.

Dr. Vijaya Nair

Table of Contents

Chapter One
The Ravages of Inflammation

> *"Inflammation may well turn out to be the elusive Holy Grail of medicine – the single phenomenon that holds the key to sickness and health."*
> *-William Joel Meggs, M.D., Ph.D., author of The Inflammation Cure (2004)*

Despite growing up in Southeast Asia, my academic schooling was firmly rooted in Western science. So, like any Western doctor, I believed that every disease had its own unique cause and required its own unique solution. Cancer happened when normal cells mutated and then developed into tumors. The solution was to poison all cells, abnormal and normal, with chemotherapy and radiation. Heart attacks occurred when a blood clot blocked the flow of blood to the heart. The solution was invasive surgery that cut through the ribcage and into the chest cavity to rearrange the blood vessels. Alzheimer's disease occurred when abnormal cell-killing structures developed in the brain. The solution was pharmaceutical drugs with side effects like nausea, vomiting, and ironically, confusion.

But in the late 1990's, everything I knew about disease was turned upside down. Study after study came out showing that the world's most feared diseases all had one thing in common – inflammation. The implications of this discovery were enormous. If inflammation was at the heart of cancer, cardiovascular disease, arthritis, digestive tract diseases, macular degeneration, Alzheimer's disease, and chronic fatigue syndrome, then instead of having to solve seven problems suddenly we only had to solve one. If we understood the unifying thread behind these debilitating diseases, alleviating their painful effects could become easy, direct, affordable, and available to most people.

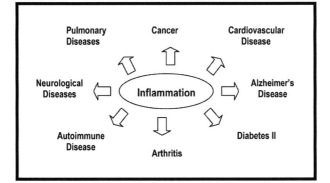

Inflammation can affect us all. If you're in good health now, managing inflammation could be your ticket to a disease-free future. If you're currently struggling with an inflammation-related disease, lowering levels of inflammation in your body will not only increase the quality of your day-to-day life, it may even extend your lifespan.

What is inflammation?

If you've ever stubbed your toe or gotten a splinter, you're familiar with the telltale signs of inflammation: redness, heat, swelling, and pain. But, did you know that inflammation can happen on the inside of your body too? Even though you can't see it, inflammation can eat away at your blood vessels, your digestive tract, your brain, your joints, and the inner structures of your eyes.

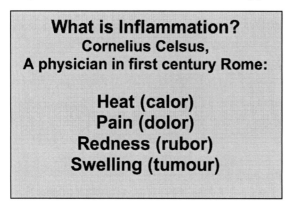

What is Inflammation?
Cornelius Celsus,
A physician in first century Rome:

Heat (calor)
Pain (dolor)
Redness (rubor)
Swelling (tumour)

Inflammation is a double-edged sword. On the one hand, it protects you. When you get a splinter, inflammation makes sure that immune cells arrive at the scene of the injury to kill any bacteria or viruses that may have entered the broken skin. That's what all that redness, heat, swelling, and pain is about. Your immune system is going to war! On the other hand, inflammation can kill you. It can cause diseases no one wants to get, like cancer, arthritis, heart disease, digestive tract diseases, macular degeneration, Alzheimer's disease, and chronic fatigue syndrome.

So when is inflammation good and when is it bad? The simple answer is that short-term inflammation is good and long-term inflammation is bad.

Enemy #1: NF-kB

At the heart of all inflammation-related diseases is nuclear factor-kappaB (or NF-kB for short.) NF-kB is a protein that plays a key role in initiating inflammation by turning certain genes on or off. NF-kB isn't inherently bad, because it protects you from infection. But if NF-kB is constantly

Deorukhkar A, et al. Back to basics: How natural products can provide the basis for new therapeutics. Expert Opin Investig Drugs. 2007;16(11):1753-1773.
Kumar A, et al. Nuclear factor-kappa B: its role in health and disease. J Mol Med. 2004 Jul;82(7):434-48.

activated, it can turn against you. When you wake this sleeping giant, it turns on over 200 genes that wreak havoc in your body. Inflammation gets turned on. Your ability to kill abnormal cells gets turned off. You become resistant to insulin, which puts you at greater risk for obesity and diabetes. And much, much more — all because this one little protein got activated.

When you have cancer, NF-kB is being activated. When you have heart disease, NF-kB is being activated. When you have AIDS, Alzheimer's, asthma, arthritis, inflammatory bowel disease, diabetes, gut diseases, lupus, multiple sclerosis, muscular dystrophy, neuropathological diseases, renal diseases, sepsis, skin diseases... NF-kB is being activated. So the key to halting inflammation — and preventing these chronic and sometimes fatal diseases — is to turn down NF-kB. You don't want to shut it off completely, because you need some inflammation. But you do want to balance it. What excites me is that natural products actually do as good a job, or better, as pharmaceuticals at turning down NF-kB!

Inflammation can be compared to firefighters battling a house on fire. They're supposed to arrive at the scene, turn their hoses on full force, put

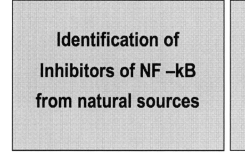

out the fire, and then go home. The house will sustain some water damage, but at least it will still be standing at the end of the day. But what would happen if, once the fire was out, the firefighters kept on spraying the house? What if they kept their hoses on for days or months or years? Eventually they would destroy the house.

Like firefighters, inflammation is only supposed to stick around as long as a threat exists. That's why your inflammation levels shoot through the roof if you have a severe bacterial infection. But, quickly go back to normal once the bacteria is successfully eliminated.[3] When the body doesn't turn off the inflammation response — when all those inflammatory chemicals stay in the system for a long time — it ends up destroying the very tissues and organs it was meant to protect. Having high levels of inflammation for short periods of time is helpful, but having low levels of inflammation for long periods of time is deadly.

Terminology to describe inflammation of various body parts

arthro = joint
arthritis = inflamed joints
broncho = bronchial tube
bronchitis = inflammation of the bronchial tubes
cardiac=heart
carditis = inflammation of the heart
cerebro=brain
cerebritis = inflammation of the brain
choleo = gallbladder
cholecystitis = inflamed gallbladder
conjunctiva = outer lining of the eye
conjunctivitis = inflammation of the outer lining of the eye
dermis = skin
dermatitis = inflamed skin
gastric = stomach
gastritis = inflammation of the lining of the stomach
hepato = liver

hepatitis = inflammation of the liver
myo = muscle
myositis = inflamed muscle
nephro = kidney
nephritis = inflamed kidney
neuro = nerve
neuritis = inflamed nerves
osteo = bone
osteitis = inflamed bones
periodontal = gums
periodontitis = inflamed gums
pneumo = lung
pneumonitis = inflamed lung
salpingo = fallopian tubes
salpingitis = inflamed fallopian tubes
vagina = vagina
vaginitis = inflammation of the vagina
vascular = blood vessel
vasculitis = inflamed blood vessels

Source: Meggs, William Joel; Svec, Carol, The Inflammation Cure.
McGraw-Hill: New York, 2004.

What triggers chronic inflammation?
So what exactly causes the immune system to go haywire? What triggers chronic inflammation? No one knows for sure, but scientists have some good theories.

One of the major suspects behind chronic, low-grade inflammation is chronic, low-grade infection. When you get a cold, food poisoning or yeast infection, your immune system goes into inflammation overdrive to protect you from the invading germs. Once the threat is conquered, inflammation goes back down to normal levels. But, what happens when the virus or bacteria or fungus doesn't completely go away? What if small amounts of it hang around in your system for months or even years? Then, instead of launching a short-lived all-out attack, the body settles for continual low-grade inflammation.

Chronic infection and chronic diseases go hand in hand. One study found that a shocking 85 percent of heart attack sufferers had chronic gum disease, which is caused by a bacterial infection.[4] People who've had three or more urinary tract infections in their lifetime have double the risk of developing bladder cancer.[5] And folks who are infected with *Heliobacter pylori* (the bacterium that causes ulcers) are six times more likely to get stomach cancer than healthy folks.[6] In all of these cases, a bacterial infection causes inflammation, and inflammation causes disease.

Other suspected causes of chronic, low-grade inflammation include smoking, air pollution, elevated levels of LDL (bad) cholesterol, high blood pressure, diets high in sugars and bad fats (both saturated and trans fats), and lack of exercise. Even emotional stress can set off the inflammatory response. A fascinating four-year study found that people who felt chronically lonely had inflammation levels two to three times as high as people who felt connected to friends and family.[7] Age is another factor. The older we get, the more pro-inflammatory chemicals our bodies produce.[8]

How inflammation causes cancer
No one wants to get cancer. There's something indescribably awful about knowing your cells are multiplying out of control and feeling helpless to do anything about it. And the conventional treatments for cancer are downright toxic. They don't distinguish between cancer cells and healthy cells — they just kill them all. Many times, the side effects of these toxic medications are so severe they actually kill the patient, or at least cause them extreme suffering.

One of my life's goals has been to help cancer patients fight their best fight against the disease. And just as important, I want to help people who are cancer-free now stay cancer-free in the future. That way you'll never have to go through the debilitating effects of chemotherapy and radiation. Whether you are fighting cancer now, or want to prevent it, here's what you need to know. Colon cancer, stomach cancer, esophageal cancer, lung cancer, liver cancer, breast cancer, cervical cancer, ovarian cancer, prostate cancer, and pancreatic cancer have *all* been linked to inflammation. This is great news, because it means that cancer doesn't just strike out of nowhere. It's preventable!

So how does cancer start? The first stage in cancer development is when a normal cell mutates into a precancerous cell. Any number of things can cause a cell to mutate, including chronic inflammation, toxic chemicals, viruses, UV radiation, or aging.

But just because you have a mutated cell doesn't mean you'll get cancer. If the body is working according to plan, it will seek out and destroy the mutated cell. Or, the mutated cell may sit dormant until some trigger (often the same inflammatory trigger that caused the mutation in the first place) causes it to change from a harmless deformed cell into a harmful malignant one. It's at this stage that the abnormal cell starts multiplying and forming a tumor. In the final stage of cancer development, the tumor gets larger and larger.

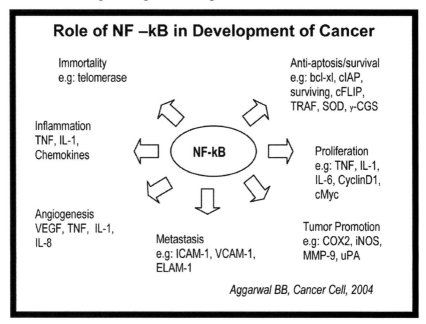

Role of NF –kB in Development of Cancer

Immortality
e.g: telomerase

Anti-aptosis/survival
e.g: bcl-xl, cIAP,
surviving, cFLIP,
TRAF, SOD, γ-CGS

Inflammation
TNF, IL-1,
Chemokines

NF-kB

Proliferation
e.g: TNF, IL-1,
IL-6, CyclinD1,
cMyc

Angiogenesis
VEGF, TNF, IL-1,
IL-8

Metastasis
e.g: ICAM-1, VCAM-1,
ELAM-1

Tumor Promotion
e.g: COX2, iNOS,
MMP-9, uPA

Aggarwal BB, Cancer Cell, 2004

All types of inflammation can cause cancer. Lung cancer can be caused by chronic smoke-induced inflammation. Esophageal cancer can be caused by acid reflux-induced inflammation. Stomach cancer can be caused by *H. pylori* (the bacterium that causes ulcers)-induced inflammation. Bladder cancer can be caused by urinary tract infection-induced inflammation. Liver cancer can be caused by hepatitis B or C-induced inflammation. Lymphoma can be caused by Epstein Barr (the virus that causes mononucleosis) -induced inflammation. Cervical cancer can be caused by *Human papillomavirus* (the virus that causes genital warts)-induced inflammation. Kidney cancer can be caused by kidney stone-induced inflammation. And colon cancer can be caused by irritable bowel syndrome-induced inflammation. Whether the inflammation is caused by an infection (such as hepatitis), a mechanical irritant (such as kidney stones), or a chemical irritant (such as stomach acid), the result is the same. Chronic, low-grade inflammation greatly increases your risk of developing cancer.

How inflammation destroys your joints

Arthritis is much more common than once thought. In the United States, one out of every three adults suffers from arthritis or other chronic joint problems.[9] If you don't have arthritis yourself, you probably know someone who does. You can seen how it could keep you from doing the things you love, like picking up a grandchild or riding a bike, thus ultimately stripping away your independence.

If you go to a Western trained medical doctor complaining of arthritic pain, chances are he or she will put you on pain killers. Unfortunately, these medications are well established to cause all kinds of side effects — including death! Aspirin and ibuprofen can cause bleeding of the stomach.[10, 11] Acetaminophen can cause liver damage.[12] And prescription pain killers such as Vioxx and Bextra were pulled from the market because they significantly increased the risk of heart attack.[13, 14] Even Celebrex, which was touted as the safe alternative to Vioxx and Bextra, has been shown to increase the risk of heart attack two-fold.[15] Yet, it's still on the market today!

Most people don't believe arthritis can be prevented because there's a common perception that joint cartilage (the cushioning that covers the bones in a joint) simply wears away with age. I know this not to be true. Joint cartilage wears away with inflammation. And if you can prevent inflammation you can prevent arthritis. Even if you already have arthritis reducing the amount of inflammation in your system will help relieve your symptoms and give you more freedom of movement — sometimes within weeks or days.

Highly movable joints such as the wrists, fingers, shoulders, hips, and knees, are the most likely to be affected by osteoarthritis. These are called "synovial joints" because the two bones meeting in this type of joint are bathed in synovia, a clear fluid whose job is to provide lubrication. Sometimes, though, the membrane that secretes the synovia becomes inflamed. Then, an avalanche of inflammatory chemicals gets released — and those inflammatory chemicals wear away the joint cartilage. The first step in any program to combat arthritis then isn't to stop the pain. It's to stop the inflammation!

How inflammation damages your heart

Your heart is the engine that keeps you going. It's your most important organ because it's what pumps blood and life-sustaining oxygen to all your other organs. So when your heart is at risk your whole body is at risk.

What's so scary about a heart attack is that it can sneak up on you from seemingly out of the blue. One day you could be feeling fine going about your day-to-day business. The next day you could be undergoing triple bypass surgery — a procedure that is incredibly invasive and from which it takes months to heal. But heart disease is not a mystery! We have the information we need right now to prevent most heart attacks.

Consider the risk factors. People with high levels of LDL cholesterol are more likely to develop cardiovascular disease. So are people who smoke and have high blood pressure; so are people who don't exercise and people who have gum disease. By now, you should know that all of these things are inflammation triggers. Cardiovascular disease is inextricably linked to inflammation. Chronic, low-grade inflammation contributes to cardiovascular disease in two ways. First, it's involved in the accumulation of plaque (or gunk) on the artery walls. Second, it causes those plaques to burst, tearing them away from the artery wall so they set sail into the bloodstream.[16] When a loose plaque creates a dam in an artery, the heart's oxygen supply is cut off, causing a heart attack.

While LDL cholesterol is still an important risk factor for cardiovascular disease, researchers are becoming increasingly convinced that C-reactive protein (CRP) (an indicator of chronic body-wide inflammation) is even more telling. According to the American Heart Association, a normal CRP reading is between 1.0 - 3.0 mg/L. If your CRP reading is just slightly elevated, at 3.0 mg/L or more, your risk of cardiovascular disease triples![17] On the other end of the spectrum, people with CRP levels below 1.0 mg/L have a low risk of developing cardiovascular disease.[18] And folks who manage to keep their CRP levels below 0.5 mg/L hardly ever have heart attacks.[19] If you want to prevent a heart attack, manage your inflammation.

How inflammation affects your digestive tract

While not life-threatening like cancer or heart disease, inflammatory bowel disease (IBD) is not something you want to get. The main types of IBD are ulcerative colitis that is typified by inflammation and ulcers in the inner lining of the large intestine, and Crohn's disease, characterized by inflammation throughout the layers of the small and/or large intestines, not just the inner lining. Crohn's disease causes abdominal pain, diarrhea, and rectal bleeding. Ulcerative colitis creates ulcers, or painful sores, in the lining of the large intestine, which bleed and produce pus.

Conventional medicine's treatment for these two painful diseases is to prescribe powerful drugs like corticosteroids. Corticosteroids may provide rapid relief of symptoms. However, because they have so many side effects they can only be used for a short amount of time. These drugs may even suppress your immunity making it harder for you to fight off infection[20] (And ironically, infection causes inflammation).

Western medicine's "cure" for ulcerative colitis is to surgically remove the colon. If you have this kind of surgery you have to wear a pouch taped to your abdomen, into which the feces drain for the rest of your life. Crohn's disease can't be cured with surgery. However, removing dysfunctional parts of the bowel is commonplace among patients with this condition.

We know that both Crohn's disease and ulcerative colitis involve inflammation of the digestive tract. But do the diseases cause the inflammation, or does the inflammation cause the diseases? No one knows for certain, but the latest thinking is that the inflammation comes first. In the case of ulcerative colitis, researchers believe a chronic viral or bacterial infection leads to on-going, low-grade inflammation of the intestinal wall.[21] In the case of Crohn's disease, the most widely accepted theory is that the immune system continually overreacts to something benign, such as foods or other foreign substances, releasing a slew of inflammatory chemicals to fight an imaginary threat.[22]

To me, it's no coincidence that IBD is more common in the United States and Europe where we eat diets higher in pro-inflammatory foods, than in less developed parts of the world. Especially when you consider that both areas have seen a dramatic increase in the incidence of IBD since the early 1950's, just when processed foods were introduced into the food supply.[23] Imagine if we could prevent these painful diseases just by managing our day-to-day inflammation levels. I think we can!

How inflammation robs you of your eyesight

What do you think the leading cause of blindness among adults over 55 in the United States and other developed countries is? Glaucoma? Cataracts? No, actually it's macular degeneration. Its prevalence is expected to increase 50 percent in the US to nearly three million people by the year 2020.[24]

Macular degeneration is a serious eye disease that slowly destroys your central vision, making things like reading, watching a movie, or driving impossible. Having macular degeneration is like having a hole in the middle of your vision. If you're looking directly at someone, you may see their hair and neck, but not their face.

Once macular degeneration has done its damage it may be impossible to bring your vision back. Therefore, the key is prevention... prevention... prevention. And yes, it can be prevented!

Similar to arthritis, macular degeneration used to be considered a disease of aging—a simple case of certain structures of the eye wearing out until vision became impaired. But new information points to inflammation as a key factor in the development and progression of this eye-ravaging disease.

Quite recently, researchers discovered that people who have a mutant version of a certain gene are 700 percent more likely to develop macular degeneration than those with the normal variety.[25] That's extremely relevant because this gene helps regulate inflammation.[26] And remember CRP, the marker for body-wide inflammation? It turns out that it's not just a predictor for heart disease. People with macular degeneration who also have high levels of CRP, have double the risk of progressing from the early and intermediate stage of the disease to the advanced stage within five years.[27]

How inflammation hurts your brain

Is there any disease more heart breaking than Alzheimer's? Can you imagine becoming so disoriented that you can no longer participate in normal conversations, or recognize the faces of people you love?

Alzheimer's disease is characterized by the development of two abnormal structures in the brain — plaques and tangles — that damage and kill nerve cells. Guess what causes those structures to develop? Inflammatory chemicals produced by your own body are the culprits.

Once again, CRP levels point to the link between inflammation and Alzheimer's. Researchers with the Honolulu-Asia Aging Study measured the CRP levels of over one thousand men from 1968-1970 and followed up with them twenty-five years later to see who developed dementia (including Alzheimer's). Compared with men who had the lowest CRP levels, men with higher levels were three times more likely to have dementia.[28]

Not only does inflammation play a role in the development of Alzheimer's. It also makes it progress faster. That's because the plaques and tangles themselves are mechanical irritants to the brain. And the inflammation they create causes the release of brain-killing chemicals.

If inflammation causes or helps cause, Alzheimer's, then anti-inflammatory drugs such as statins, (commonly used to treat high cholesterol) should reduce the risk of developing the disease. Indeed they do — dramatically. Research shows people who take statins are up to 70 percent less likely to get Alzheimer's than those who don't.[29] But don't rush to your doctor to get a prescription for statins — there is a natural, safer, more effective and more economical way to prevent the disease as we will reveal in the following chapters.

How inflammation reduces your energy
In our modern culture where everyone seems intent on accomplishing more things in less time, feeling fatigue isn't the exception — it's the rule. Would it surprise you to learn that your lack of energy could be directly related to the amount of inflammation in your body?

Think about the last time you were sick – really sick; so sick that you couldn't work. How did you feel? How was your energy level? Did you find it difficult to do anything more than lie around on the couch watching movies all day? If so, you've had a direct experience with inflammation-related fatigue.

As you may remember, inflammation is a response of the immune system to a foreign invader. So when you're fighting a cold or flu, your immune system is releasing high levels of inflammatory chemicals to beat off the bad guys. Those chemicals also have an effect on your brain making you feel drained of energy. This is a built-in evolutionary response of the body — as long as you're on the couch, your immune system can devote all of its energy to fighting the infection.

People who are chronically tired may be exhausted because their bodies have been battling a low-grade infection for months, or even years. Eventually that kind of chronic, low-grade inflammation takes its toll. Unfortunately, Western medicine doesn't have much to offer people who feel drained day in and day out. Doctors may advise you to get more sleep, eat a healthy diet, and start a mild exercise program — all sound advice. But sometimes even with lifestyle changes, the lack of energy doesn't go away. Your doctor might then recommend that you see a mental health professional (as if the fatigue is all in your head), or take antidepressants (as if the depression is making you fatigued rather than the fatigue making you depressed). This advice does not address the true source of the problem — and may make it worse.[30]

But if your fatigue is caused by a low-level infection, you need to kill the germs to get to the root of the problem. Luckily you don't have to take antibiotics, which rid the body of all bacteria — both bad and good. You can take an herb that is both antimicrobial and gentle instead.

Chapter Two
The Importance of Antioxidants

> "Inflammation is the evil twin of oxidation.
> Where you find one, you find the other."
> *-James Joseph, neuroscientist, Tufts University (2005)*

No doubt you've heard of antioxidants. You know they're good for you. You may even know why — because they combat harmful free radicals (unstable molecules that damage our cellular DNA). But, did you know that antioxidants also play a key role in combating inflammation?

What are antioxidants?
To understand what an antioxidant is first you have to understand what an oxidant is. An oxidant is a substance that steals an electron from another molecule through a reaction with oxygen. You've seen oxidation happen before. A bicycle exposed to oxygen in the form of rainwater, rusts. An apple exposed to oxygen in the form of air turns brown. And human cells exposed to oxygen in the form of oxidants (also known as free radicals), become damaged.

Free radicals are like parasites. These predator molecules are missing an electron, which makes them hungry for a new one. Just as parasites need to steal resources from a human host to survive free radicals need to steal electrons from healthy cells to survive, which damages the cells' DNA. Unfortunately, every cell that is the victim of a free radical attack becomes a free radical itself. And so the cycle of damage continues.

Antioxidants are substances that prevent oxidation. In a selfless act of sacrifice, they donate electrons to the parasite free radicals so they don't come after human cells. By stabilizing the free radicals antioxidants stop the cycle of damage.

How oxidation contributes to disease
It's now commonly accepted that free radicals are the main cause of aging in the human body. The free radical theory of aging is described as follows: Oxidation damages human cells. When a cell sustains enough damage it dies. And when enough of a person's cells are damaged or killed, they age. Free radical damage, also called "oxidative stress," has been linked to many diseases including cardiovascular disease, cancer,

arthritis, eye diseases, and Alzheimer's disease.

So what causes oxidation? There are many contributing factors. Some are unavoidable, such as breathing and digestion. But others are within our control, like smoking, alcohol consumption, emotional stress, and diets high in sugars and bad fats (both saturated and trans fats). Do you notice a connection? All of these things are also inflammation triggers.

The connection between inflammation and oxidation

If free radicals are so destructive then why does the body produce them? The answer is simple – free radicals are a necessary evil, a byproduct of normal metabolism. In an ideal world they aren't a problem because they're neutralized by antioxidants produced by the body. But, we don't live in an ideal world. Most of us are exposed to far more free radicals through our modern lifestyles than our bodies were ever designed to handle. Compounding the problem is the fact that we eat far fewer antioxidant-rich foods (such as fruits and vegetables) than our bodies were meant to. The fundamental problem then is we have too many free radicals and not enough antioxidants.

Free radicals aren't all bad. In fact, they're an important part of the immune response. When germs enter your body your immune system unleashes an army of destructive agents to kill them — including the free radicals. For example, if you get food poisoning from eating a medium-rare hamburger tainted with E. coli, your immune system creates free radicals on purpose to kill the bacteria. In addition to their role as hired guns, free radicals also call on inflammatory chemicals as back-up to help battle the germs. Therefore, oxidation causes inflammation. In the short-term, all that oxidation and inflammation is a good thing. But if your poor body is subjected to those forces continually they won't just damage the "bad guys," they'll damage the parts of the body they were called in to rescue.

A good example of this phenomenon in action is the development of atherosclerosis, or the accumulation of plaque within the arteries. High levels of cholesterol have been considered the major cause of atherosclerosis and people with high LDL cholesterol would be at greater risk of developing the condition. But, a shocking 50 percent of people who have heart attacks do not have elevated cholesterol! Now scientists are realizing the problem isn't cholesterol per sé – it's oxidized cholesterol, which is cholesterol that has been attacked by free radicals because the body didn't have enough antioxidants to protect itself.

Oxidized cholesterol doesn't look right to the immune system.

So what does it do? It launches an attack against it, complete with an army of inflammatory chemicals and white blood cells! And unfortunately, the inflammation damages the arterial walls and contributes to the development of plaque, causing atherosclerosis. Researchers who tested the theory that oxidized cholesterol initiates atherosclerosis got very interesting results. When mice were fed a diet containing oxidized cholesterol, their development of fatty streak lesions (the first sign of atherosclerosis) was accelerated by up to 38 percent.

So in a nutshell, what's the link between inflammation and oxidation? The body produces free radicals in response to a threat. Free radicals cause oxidation. Oxidation causes inflammation. And inflammation causes damage. By neutralizing free radicals, antioxidants prevent oxidation — and therefore quell inflammation.

If you had told me fifteen years ago that today I would be authoring a book about natural anti-inflammatory remedies for combating major diseases, I probably wouldn't have believed you. Because of my conventional Western medical background I was skeptical of reports of chronically and terminally ill patients who, using complementary and alternative medicines, were experiencing significant improvements in their quality of life.

PREVENT CANCER

Chapter Three
My Top Seven Natural Anti-Inflammatory & Antioxidant Supplements

"The chemical diversity, structural complexity, affordability, lack of substantial toxic effects and inherent biological activity of natural products makes them ideal candidates for new therapeutics."
-Amir Deorukhkar, Sunil Krishnan, Gautam Sethi, & Bharat B. Aggarwal, researchers at The University of Texas MD Anderson Cancer Center (2007)

After almost a decade of reviewing studies conducted by scientists and academicians at distinguished universities and institutions on three continents, as well as performing my own independent research, I can now say that natural remedies present exciting methods for treating and preventing a range of debilitating diseases. This chapter covers my top seven natural anti-inflammatory and antioxidant supplements to help you prevent and even treat, some of the world's most feared diseases.

Much has been written about possible adverse side effects resulting from the excessive ingestion of soy-based products. Some of this information is accurate "if" the author is writing only about uncultured soy. Thus, it is absolutely critical that one understands the difference between scientifically cultured soy and the uncultured soy that is found in most products that contain soy. To compare the two is like comparing apples and oranges. All references in this book are to "cultured" or properly fermented soy that has been scientifically formulated in a way that is evidence-based and therapeutic to the human body.

1. Cultured Soy and Cancer

Americans are eating more soybean products than ever before. Soy is showing up everywhere — in fortified juices, imitation meats, dairy-free cheeses, yogurts, and frozen desserts; nutrition bars, cereals; and more. It makes sense. After all, soy is the only complete food in the botanical kingdom. It contains 42 percent protein, more than any other plant.[36] It's high in fiber. It's a natural source of good-for-you omega-3 fatty acids. It's a powerhouse of protective antioxidants and phyto-nutrients (beneficial compounds found in plants). It provides a wealth of vitamins, including vitamins A (as beta-carotene), B^1, B^2, B^{12}, C, D, E, and K — and several essential minerals, such as selenium and zinc. And mounting evidence shows it may prevent cancer.

But, there's a catch. *In order to reap the nutritional and anti-cancer benefits of soy, it must be cultured.* Culturing simply means adding beneficial microbial cultures to a food and letting them transform it into something more nutritious and digestible. Yogurt, sour cream, kefir, and pickles are all examples of cultured foods.

The importance of culturing

If you take a trip to China, Japan, Indonesia, or Singapore, you'll find that the traditional Asian diet does not include large quantities of super-processed, genetically modified soy products like we have in Western countries today (such as isolated soy protein, a common ingredient found in nutrition bars). It incorporates small amounts of natural, *cultured* whole soy foods, such as natto (cultured soybeans), miso (a condiment made from cultured soybean paste), shoyu (soy sauce or tamari), and tempeh (a compact cultured soybean cake). In fact, soy wasn't even considered edible until fermentation techniques were developed during the Chou Dynasty.[37]

What the producers of modern, uncultured soy foods won't tell you is that in addition to all the nutrients it contains, soy also contains *anti-nutrients*. These anti-nutrients prevent your body from absorbing essential minerals and trace elements. Unfortunately, cooking will not destroy these anti-nutrients. Only the culturing process will.

Another benefit of culturing is that it makes it easier for your body to digest and absorb the goodness of soy. When you culture a food, you're basically using beneficial microbial cultures to pre-digest it. Those cultures transform large, hard-to-digest molecules into small, easy-to-digest ones. Not only that, culturing soy also reduces its allergic qualities. (Soy is one of the most common food allergens.) According to two newly published research papers, tests in samples of human blood showed that when soy is cultured, its potential to produce an allergic reaction is reduced by as much as 99 percent.[38]

The most important benefit of culturing, though, is that the process is thought to convert certain phyto-nutrients, called genistein and daidzin, into their active anti-cancer forms, genistein and daidzein. Both genistein and daidzein are powerful antioxidant and anti-inflammatory agents that have been shown in voluminous laboratory studies to work in multiple ways against cancer.

Whole soy vs. isolated soy phyto-nutrients

If genistein and daidzein are so great, why not just take those specific phyto-nutrients in pill form? The answer lies in the old adage "the whole is greater than the sum of its parts." Individually, genistein and daidzein are soy's most powerful anti-carcinogenic constituents. However, soybeans contain *numerous* cancer-fighting compounds that work synergistically. One of the most important principles of traditional herbal medicine is that it is the whole herb (or whole soybean in this case) that's important — not isolated fractions.

In fact, research has shown that soy, with the anti-carcinogenic iso-flavones genistein and daidzein removed, was more effective at shrinking tumors than those phyto-nutrients by themselves.[39] In other words, genistein and daidzein are only part of the complete picture of whole soy.

My interest in cultured soy

I have a special interest in the healing power of cultured soy. As earlier mentioned, I was raised in Singapore, an island nation in Southeast Asia. About 75 percent of the population of Singapore is ethnically Chinese. Therefore, growing up I had friends whose parents ran traditional Chinese medicine shops that sold cultured soy foods.

Because of my childhood familiarity with these foods, as an adult I was particularly intrigued when I heard about some of the fantastic results people with terminal cancer were experiencing from drinking 8 ounces. a day of a liquid cultured soy beverage. However, because of my Western scientific training, I had to see factual evidence to be convinced that this treatment could be of value.

While at Columbia University, I came upon some promising research on cultured soy that showed it was extremely effective as a nutritional supplement for malnutrition, especially in people with terminal cancers and chronic infections. Knowing that this information could revolutionize modern cancer therapy, I decided cultured soy was worthy of investigation.

For six years, I worked with various centers across the globe studying cultured soy, as well as documenting the incredible response of individual cancer patients to the treatment through biopsies, blood tests, and patients' own evaluations of how cultured soy improved their symptoms. The case reports I compiled won recognition from the Office of Cancer Complementary and Alternative Medicine (OCCAM) at the National Cancer Institute. Based on that initial groundwork, there is now a human clinical study being conducted at The University of Texas, MD Anderson Cancer Center using cultured soy to treat the complications of cancer. As of this printing, that study is not yet completed, but I can share with you the research that first got my attention back in 2001. And I can also share what I observed working one on one with terminal cancer patients who were lucky enough to be introduced to cultured soy.

What cultured soy research says

Research shows that cultured soy can be used both as a cancer preventative and treatment. On the prevention side, a mountain of evidence shows that populations who eat soy regularly (primarily in the form of cultured soy) have lower rates of breast cancer, lung cancer, prostate cancer, and leukemia.[40] A 2002 study of Asian-American women, for example, found that those who ate four servings of soy a week (including cultured soy foods such as miso and natto) during adolescence and adulthood slashed their risk of developing breast cancer in half.[41] And a 2007 study of Japanese men showed that those with the highest intake of genistein and daidzien through consuming soy (again, including cultured soy foods such as miso and natto) were 58 percent less likely to develop prostate cancer than those with the lowest intake.[42] If you want to prevent cancer, it just makes sense to include a little cultured soy in your diet every day.

What excites me most, however, is cultured soy's effect on people who have already developed cancer. The most impressive study to date was a human clinical trial conducted at six different hospitals and one medical school in China. A total of 318 patients with 23 different kinds of cancer participated in the study, all of who were receiving either chemotherapy or radiation. About two-thirds of the patients were given a cultured soy beverage daily, while the other third, which acted as the "control" or comparison group, received a standard medical preparation.

After six months, *over 90 percent* of the people in the cultured soy group experienced improvements in their quality of life, such as a noticeable increase in the amount of energy they felt. Their immune function improved. And they experienced fewer side effects from the chemotherapy and radiation treatments, such as decreased appetite, nausea, and vomiting.[43]

These results are very similar to what I have observed first-hand working with cancer patients. Time and time again, I saw that patients undergoing chemotherapy and radiation treatments (which are somewhat effective against certain cancers but can have devastating side effects) experienced tremendous improvement in the way they felt once they started taking cultured soy. People who were terminally ill, who had been given just a few months to live, were picking up their lives and actually going back to work! In addition to improving people's quality of life, I also observed that cultured soy helped reduce the amount of cancer in terminally ill patients'. How? By making sure their bodies didn't become resistant to the conventional therapies.

One of the drawbacks of chemotherapy and radiation is that they increase the activity of the pro-inflammatory protein NF-kB, and make cancer cells less sensitive to cell-killing agents. When that happens, the patient may become "chemo-resistant" or "radiation-resistant," meaning he or she stops responding to the therapy.

What's so amazing about cultured soy is that it turns down the pro-inflammatory protein that causes treatment resistance. After taking cultured soy for six months my case study patients, who were once resistant to chemotherapy or radiation, started responding again. This is very exciting for scientists because once a patient develops resistance to chemotherapy or radiation, it's pretty much the end of the road — there's nothing much you can do. If there is a natural product that can reverse that state, it may bring hope to those who are suffering.

But cultured soy doesn't just make chemo and radiation work better; it also has antitumor properties of its own. Being a firm believer in complementary medicine, which advocates a combination of Western and Eastern healing therapies, I would never suggest that a cancer patient solely choose cultured soy to the exclusion of conventional treatment, rather I'd advise them to use it as an adjunct therapy. However, some of the individuals I studied did make the choice to use each in conjunction with the other, and the results were nothing short of extraordinary!

One of the case reports I submitted to OCCAM tracked a 67-year-old woman who was diagnosed with breast cancer in August of 1997. She had a tumor that was 15 x 15 x 20 mm in size. It was recommended that she have a total mastectomy or lumpectomy with removal of the auxiliary lymph nodes, followed by aggressive radiation and hormonal treatment. However, she refused all standard therapy. The doctors gave her six months to live. The woman began taking a cultured soy beverage in November of 1997 and received regular mammograms. Gradually the tumor decreased in size, until by January of 2001, it was just 7 x 5 x 6 mm. In February of 2004 — six years after she was supposed to have died — her mammogram and ultrasound readings did not show any evidence of malignant lesions. She is still alive and well today.

Mark N. Mead, MSc, Integrative Nutrition & Wellness Coaching, Carolina Center for Integrative Medicine, Associate Editor of "Integrative Cancer Therapies," and co-author of *The Rapid Recovery Handbook* comments: "In my work as a nutritional oncology specialist, I have been consistently impressed with cultured soy and curcumin in terms of their ability to enhance the quality of life for people undergoing cancer treatment and those in recovery. I have known a number of individuals with advanced cancers who have gone on to surprise their oncologists by substantially exceeding all statistically based expectations for survival."

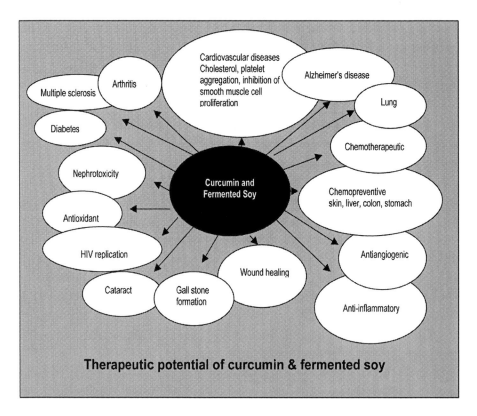

Therapeutic potential of curcumin & fermented soy

2. Curcumin and arthritis

While I was busy studying cultured soy, a noted and renowned researcher, Dr. Bharat B. Aggarwal, was doing groundbreaking work with curcumin (pronounced kir-KYOO-min). Even if you've never heard of curcumin, you've probably eaten it before. Curcumin is the major constituent of turmeric. It's what gives the spice its characteristic yellow-orange color. But turmeric does more than just add flavor and color to curries. It's been used in Traditional Chinese Medicine and the ancient Indian medical system called Ayurveda (pronounced are-yu-VAY-duh) for thousands of years to treat a variety of inflammatory diseases. The work of Dr. Aggarwal and other scientists over the past decade has confirmed curcumin's ability to fight inflammation, which is one reason why it has become a popular natural remedy for arthritis.

What curcumin research says

Research has shown curcumin is a powerful antioxidant that is ten times more active than vitamin E.[44] It's also a potent anti-inflammatory with efficacy rivaling that of both cortisone and phenylbutazone.[45] How does it work? It works in many ways, but one of the primary modes is by shutting down the same pro-inflammatory protein that cultured soy shuts down.[46] In other words, curcumin tells the body to put away the fire hoses and turn the inflammation off.

A number of animal studies support curcumin's ability to relieve the pain and swelling of both osteo and rheumatoid arthritis. One study found that when curcumin was given to arthritic rats it lowered levels of an inflammatory protein by a stunning 73 percent.[47] Another study, also in rats, showed that turmeric extract profoundly curbed joint inflammation and joint destruction.[48] A study in dogs with osteoarthritis found that turmeric extract reduced lameness and joint pain.[49]

Curcumin seems to work in humans too. In a study consisting of eighteen patients with rheumatoid arthritis, after just two weeks curcumin caused significant improvements in morning stiffness, joint swelling, and walking ability.[50] Human cell studies have additionally shown that curcumin suppresses the inflammatory chemicals that contribute to the development of osteoarthritis,[51] and decreases some of the abnormal changes in joint tissue that characterizes rheumatoid arthritis. [52]

I've seen tremendous improvement in patients with arthritis who take large doses of curcumin. But, I also think it's a great tool for preventing this disease in the first place. Remember, joints don't just "wear out" with age. They wear out because of inflammation. If you can keep your inflammation levels under control with a daily dose of curcumin, you may reduce your risk of ever getting arthritis.

NIH-Funded Grants on Curcumin

Grant	Source	Investigator	Institute	Duration	Subject
RO1	NCI	S. Shrikant	Wash U	2005-9	Colon cancer
R21	NCI	J. bright	Vanderbilt	2003-6	ATL
R01	NIAID	M. Chan	Temple	1002-6	Leishmaniasis
R21	NCI	S. Gautam	Michigan	2005-6	Prostate
R01	NHLBI	S. Hoffman	US Carolina	2003-7	Scleroderma
RO1	NIDDK	P. Keila	U Arizona	2005-10	IBD
RO1	NCI	C. Koumenis	Wake Forest U	2005-9	Radio/Chemo Semsitizer
RO1	NCI	C.V. Rao	Oklahoma U	1999-6	Colon cancer
R21	NCI	M. Christofidou	U. Penn	2006-7	Radiation-induced Pneumonopathy
R03	NCI	J.C. States	U. Louisville	2005-7	BP-DNA damage
R01	NIA	G.K. Pavlath	Emory U	2001-6	Muscle atrophy
R21	NCI	J.D. Burton	CMMI-Bellville	2003-6	Chronobiological
P50	NIA	G.M. Cole	UCLA	2005	Alzheimer
R01	NCCAM	G.M. Cole	UCLA	2005-9	Alzheimer
R01	NIA	S. Frautschy	UCLA	2004-6	Alzheimer
R01	NIA	S. Frautschy	UCLA	2004-9	Neurodegeneration
R01	NCI	K.S. Lee	UNC	2005-10	Analogues
R21	NCI	S. Raj-Vadhan	UTMDACC	2004-6	Multiple Myeloma
R21	NCI	R. Kurzrock	UTMDACC	2004-6	Pancreatic cancer
R21	NCI	B. Ponnappa	Thom. Jefferson	2004-6	Liver targeting

3. Resveratrol and cardiovascular disease

How is it that the French eat a diet higher in fat than Americans, yet enjoy lower rates of cardiovascular disease? Could it be that the large amounts of red wine they regularly drink is somehow protecting their hearts? That's what many scientists believe. Found naturally in the skin of red grapes, and therefore red wine, resveratrol (pronounced ress-VAIR-uh-trawl) may hold the answer to the French Paradox. In fact, few natural substances have generated as much excitement among anti-aging researchers as this phyto-nutrient.

What research on resveratrol says

In late 2006, researchers at Harvard Medical School and the National Institute on Aging created a stir when they published a study showing that resveratrol appeared to counter the negative effects of an unhealthy diet. When mice were fed a diet very high in fat, they quickly developed the telltale signs of pre-diabetes – grossly enlarged livers, elevated blood sugar, and high levels of insulin (the hormone that escorts blood sugar into the cells). But, when mice were fed the same high-fat diet, only this time supplemented with resveratrol, they stayed just as healthy and active as mice fed a standard low-fat diet — and lived just as long! It's as if the resveratrol wiped out the negative effects of the unhealthy diet. [53]

More recently, a 2008 study found that resveratrol blocked a full 92 percent of age-related gene changes in the heart.[54] As we age, certain genes in our heart tissue switch off while others switch on. Unfortunately, those changes aren't usually good. By stopping those age-related gene changes, resveratrol appears to keep the heart young.

And that's where things really get interesting. So far, resveratrol has been shown to increase the life spans of various forms of life — including worms, fruit flies, fish, dogs, and monkeys.[55, 56] Not many other substances can say the same, which is why resveratrol has the scientific world so excited. Will it do the same in humans? We won't know the answer to that question for some time, but I happen to know of at least one prominent resveratrol researcher who is enough of a believer that he takes it himself.

How exactly does resveratrol work? Scientists believe it acts in the same way that severe calorie restriction does. When mice eat a diet that contains 40 percent fewer calories than normal, they live longer — 50 percent longer.[57] While we don't know whether calorie restriction will have the same effect in humans, we do know that people who eat low-calorie diets benefit from lowered cholesterol and blood pressure, less body fat, and lower levels of CRP — that indicator of body-wide inflammation.[58]

Why does calorie restriction improve heart health and longevity? The theory is that animals are wired for two modes – reproduction and maintenance. They go into reproduction mode when food is abundant because the living is easy and there's enough to go around for everyone. They revert to maintenance mode when food is scarce because it becomes more important to conserve energy and fight off starvation in order to make it through the famine. It seems that resveratrol turns on the same longevity gene that calorie slashing does — without any of the sacrifices.[59]

4. Ginger and digestive health

You've probably eaten foods seasoned with ginger, or even cooked with this spicy herb yourself. I grew up eating ginger frequently because it's a common spice in Singapore. But, did you know that ginger has value as a medicinal plant? For thousands of years ginger root has played an important role in some of the world's major herbal traditions, including Traditional Chinese Medicine, Ayurveda, and Traditional European Medicine. All of these systems of medicine recognize that ginger is an excellent herb for ailments of the digestive tract, including nausea, gas, abdominal pain, diarrhea, constipation, colic, and painful digestion.[60]

How can ginger help you? It supports digestion by calming stomach contractions.[61] It prevents motion sickness (One study found it worked significantly better than Dramamine!).[62] It relieves the symptoms of morning sickness.[63] And it relieves nausea and vomiting among people who've just had surgery.[64] So if you have problems with digestion — such as gas, abdominal pains, and bloating — or if you suffer from nausea or vomiting (whether from motion sickness, pregnancy, or surgery), ginger is a great herb for you.

What the research reveals about ginger

Modern research has shown that ginger suppresses pro-inflammatory compounds and blocks the production of free radicals.[65] That makes it a powerful anti-inflammatory agent and antioxidant.

Exciting new research has uncovered that ginger is useful for more than just short-term upsets of the digestive tract. It actually turns off several genes that are responsible for chronic inflammation.[66] That means ginger holds great promise for preventing diseases associated with inflammation of the digestive tract.

Several studies in rodents have indicated ginger could be an effective treatment for inflammatory bowel disease. One study found that in mice with ulcerative colitis, ginger extract lowered levels of inflammatory compounds anywhere from 29-73 percent.[67] Another study observed that when rats with ulcerative colitis were given ginger extract, every single marker of the disease — including levels of inflammation and oxidation — improved. In fact, the effect was comparable to the pharmaceutical drug sulfasalizine.[68] The major difference is that sulfasalizine is known to *cause* gastro-intestinal disturbances — such as nausea, vomiting, and gastric distress[69] — while ginger is known to *prevent* them!

5. Lutein and macular degeneration

If you were able to magically peer into the very back of your eye, to the part that's responsible for detailed central vision, what color do you think it would be? The answer is yellow. Why? Because this tiny oval structure, called the macula, is saturated with lutein (pronounced LOO-tene), a yellow pigment found in plants.[70]

Lutein, which occurs naturally in marigolds, corn, egg yolks, spinach, broccoli, squash, and peas, plays a very special role in a plant's life. It acts like a "botanical sunscreen," protecting the plant against the harmful effects of ultraviolet light. As it turns out, lutein offers the same protection to your eyes. When you eat foods that contain lutein, the yellow pigment is deposited into the macula. There, it creates a shield that protects the macula from the damaging free radicals created by UV rays.

What the research says about Lutein

Imagine if, just by taking a little lutein pill each day, you could prevent macular degeneration — the leading cause of blindness among adults over 55 in the United States and other developed countries. That's exactly what the research on lutein is showing.

Numerous studies have concluded that the more lutein you ingest, the less likely you are to develop this eye-destroying disease. The most recent study, which tracked nearly 2,500 people for five to ten years, found that people who got the most lutein and zeaxanthin (a sister pigment) through diet slashed their risk of developing macular degeneration by an incredible 65 percent.[71]

Even if you already have macular degeneration, lutein can help. One of the biggest human clinical trials to date on lutein, called the Lutein Antioxidant Supplementation Trial (or LAST), tracked what happened when macular degeneration patients were given lutein supplements or placebo pills for a year. Researchers found that those who took lutein experienced significant improvements in their visual acuity (sharpness of vision) and contrast sensitivity (the ability to make out objects that blend into a similarly colored background) compared to those who took a placebo.[72] Neither the researchers nor the subjects knew who was getting the dummy pill and who was getting the real thing, so there was no possibility of a "placebo effect."

Because lutein and zeaxanthin have such a profound effect on vision, some researchers have even asked if these two pigments are "conditionally essential" nutrients. In other words, while lutein and zeaxanthin don't have official vitamin or mineral status, might they be just as essential?[73] I think the answer is yes. In fact, low levels of macular lutein and zeaxanthin are now considered a risk factor for the development of macular degeneration.[74]

Unfortunately, most people in developed countries don't eat nearly the amount of fruits and vegetables needed to get optimal levels of lutein. Scientists have determined we need between 6-20 mg of this important phyto-nutrient per day to protect against macular degeneration. Yet in the United States, the mean intake is just 1.7 mg per day.[75] Not only that, levels of lutein and zeaxanthin within the macula decline with age.[76] That makes it especially important for anyone over 50 to supplement their diets with lutein.

6. Ashwaghanda and Alzheimer's disease

You've probably never heard of ashwaghanda (pronounced osh-wah-GAHN-duh), but I bet you've heard of ginseng. Ashwaghanda plays a similar role in Ayurveda to the role ginseng plays in Traditional Chinese Medicine. In fact, ashwaghanda's nickname is Indian ginseng.

For over 3,000 years, the people of India have relied on ashwaghanda to do two seemingly opposite things, energize them and relax them. Ashwaghanda belongs to a class of herbs called adaptogens, so named because they help the body adapt to whatever conditions it's facing. If you're low on energy ashwaghanda will energize you. If you're high on stress ashwaghanda will relax you. It has the amazing ability to read what your body needs and then deliver it.

Recently, researchers have been investigating ashwaghanda's potential to improve brain function in cases of dementia and what they're finding is very exciting. Dementia, also called senility, is a general term for the loss of thinking ability that happens when brain cells die. Alzheimer's disease and stroke can both cause dementia. Tragically, there is no cure for dementia. According to Western medicine it's impossible to undo damage to the brain once it's occurred. The best modern drugs can do is improve the symptoms or slow down the progression of the disease.

But what if Western science is wrong? What if there *is* a way to repair brain damage? What if a diagnosis of Alzheimer's disease no longer means a patient is doomed to lose their ability to think and speak clearly, or forget the faces of their loved ones, or become so debilitated that they can no longer take care of themselves? That's the promise of ashwaghanda.

What ashwaghanda research reveals

So far, five different studies have shown that certain phyto-nutrients in ashwaghanda can reverse brain dysfunction and improve memory in mice and rats. Not surprisingly, when rats with memory loss are put in a maze they have trouble navigating it. They can't remember where they've been. They just end up going around and around in circles. But, giving ashwaghanda extract to the rats for four weeks reverses their memory loss enabling them to navigate the maze with ease.[77] Similar memory-restorative results have been demonstrated in mice.[78, 79, 80]

How does it work? This is the part I find most fascinating. Several test tube and animal studies have discovered that ashwaghanda actually regenerates brain cells! When added to human and animal brain cell cultures, ashwaghanda extract promotes the growth of critical structures in both normal and damaged brain cells.[81,82,83,84] One study in mice found that ashwaghanda phyto-nutrients helped preserve key brain cell structures, even in the face of a brain-toxic drug.[85]

Based on this information, researchers have declared one ashwaghanda phyto-nutrient "an important candidate for the therapeutic treatment of neurodegenerative diseases, as it is able to reconstruct neuronal networks"[86] and said that another phyto-nutrient from ashwaghanda "may ameliorate dysfunction in Alzheimer's disease."[87] This is huge news. If these results translate to humans, then ashwaghanda, a simple and inexpensive herb of nature, could change the lives of millions of people in a way no drug has been able to do.

In addition to regenerating brain cells, there are two other ways ashwaghanda may improve thinking ability and restore memory. First, it appears to block the breakdown of a brain chemical responsible for learning and memory.[88, 89, 90] Second, it acts as an antioxidant, preventing the damage caused to brain cells by free radicals.[91,92]

One thing I find striking about this ancient herb is how quickly it appears to work. One study looked at mice whose ability to acquire and attain information had been disrupted by the drug scopolamine. The mice regained their brain function after just *one day* of treatment with ashwaghanda.[93]

7. Green tea and energy

Legend has it that green tea was discovered by accident. Back in 2737 B.C, the servants of Chinese emperor Shen Nung would make a fire every day to boil and sanitize his drinking water. One day, they used the branches of the *Camellia sinensis* shrub for kindling (a plant we now refer to as tea), and some stray leaves ended up in the pot. After drinking the leaf-infused beverage the emperor extolled its virtues, saying it gave "vigor of body, contentment of mind, and determination of purpose."[94] Tea cultivation became widespread in China and soon caught on in Japan.

Modern research shows Shen Nung was onto something. Study after study reveals green tea is a modern panacea that may protect against debilitating diseases such as Alzheimer's, Parkinson's, heart disease, and cancer. But I want to talk about green tea's benefits for something much simpler and that affects much more of the population: lack of energy. If you suffer from the afternoon slump, green tea is the perfect get-up-and-go energizer. It provides an even, sustained energy without the crash of artificial stimulants.

Most people think that green tea's energizing properties come from its caffeine content. But even when green tea is decaffeinated, it still has an energizing effect. Why? I think there are three reasons: its high levels of antioxidants, its ability to combat inflammation, and its anti-microbial properties.

What the research says about green tea

Thanks to green tea's content of the phyto-nutrient ECGC, it is twenty-five times stronger as an antioxidant than vitamin E, and one-hundred times stronger than vitamin C! How do antioxidants contribute to energy? Inside each of your cells is a tiny energy-generating factory called the mitochondria. Free radicals are like vandals. They attack these mini-factories and damage their machinery, impairing their ability to create energy. Antioxidants protect the mitochondria from free radicals, so they maintain the cells' energy-generating capacity.[95]

Studies in test tubes and animals have also shown that green tea has anti-inflammatory properties. What does quelling inflammation have to do with energy? As you may remember from *Chapter One*, one of the side effects of inflammation is fatigue. If your body is battling an outside invader, it needs to divert its energy away from normal metabolism and towards fighting the threat. And that makes you tired. ECGC, the powerful antioxidant contained in green tea, turns off a key gene involved in inflammation.[96] Hypothetically, that could increase your feelings of energy.

But what really peaks my interest about green tea is its potent antiviral and anti-bacterial properties. If your body is in an inflammatory state due to a chronic infection, such as periodontal disease or hepatitis, then ridding yourself of the infection should stop the inflammation — and the fatigue that goes along with it.

In test tube studies green tea has been shown to kill the following viruses or stop them from replicating: hepatitis B,[97] influenza,[98] herpes simplex type 2,[99] HIV,[100,101] adenovirus (which causes respiratory illnesses),[102] rotaviruses (which cause diarrhea among young children and infants), enteroviruses (which usually cause mild respiratory illnesses but can cause meningitis or, rarely, encephalitis),[103] and Epstein-Barr (which causes mononucleosis).[104]

Green tea has also been shown to kill a broad spectrum of bacteria, including food-borne bacteria such as *Escherichia coli*, *Salmonella Typhimurium*, *Listeria monocytogenes*, *Staphylococcus aureus*, and *Bacillus cereus*;[105] dental plaque bacteria such as *E. coli*, *Streptococcus salivarius*, and *Streptococcus mutans*;[106] diarrheal disease bacteria such as *Staphylococcus aureus*, *S. epidermidis*, *Vibrio cholera O1*, *V. cholera non O1*, *V. parahaemolyticus*, *V. mimicus*, *Campylobacter jejuni* and *Plesiomonas shigelloides*; and the ulcer-causing bacteria *Heliobacter pylori*.[107]

Granted, test tube studies are not the same as studies in real, live human beings. But if human research bears out the test tube research — if green tea can kill viruses and bacteria in humans — it could be a powerful way to fight inflammation-induced fatigue at its source. If you don't like the taste of green tea, don't worry as you can get all the benefits this botanical has to offer in capsule form. And if you're sensitive to caffeine, decaffeinated green tea is available as both a tea and a supplement.

PREVENT CANCER

Chapter Four
Why I Prefer Formulas over Single Ingredients

"Herbal formulas are developed to use each herb to its greatest advantage. By combining different herbs together, we will not only adjust and increase the treatment results, but also reduce or release the side-effects from the other herbs."

-www.acupuncture.com (2007)

East vs. West

In Western countries such as the United States and much of Europe, there is a prevailing belief that every disease has its own unique cause and requires its own unique solution. Western medicine is very good at pinpointing exactly where a physiological problem lies, and then prescribing a targeted therapy to fix the problem. The weakness of this approach is that it doesn't look at the bigger picture. For example, in its zeal to create drugs that block the exact enzyme involved in arthritis inflammation (COX-2) Western medicine overlooked the fact that COX-2 actually does good things too! When you block it completely, as was the case with Vioxx and Bextra, you end up dramatically increasing the risk for heart attack and stroke.[108, 109]

In certain Asian countries such as China and India that gave birth to some of the oldest medical systems on earth, Traditional Chinese Medicine and Ayurveda, the approach is more holistic centering on the whole body. Rather than trying to zero in on the single cause behind each disease, traditional Chinese and Ayurvedic doctors look for patterns of disharmony or imbalance. In the words of Oriental medicine doctor Ted J. Kaptchuk, "One does not ask 'What X is causing Y?' but rather, 'What is the relationship between X and Y?'"[110] The weakness of this approach is that it doesn't get into the physiology of what's actually happening at the cellular level. For example, Eastern health practitioners aren't particularly interested in NF-kB, the protein that is linked with every single one of the diseases covered in this book.

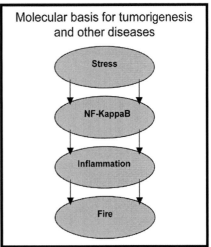

Molecular basis for tumorigenesis and other diseases

Stress

NF-KappaB

Inflammation

Fire

I think that *both* approaches have value. I tend to take a Western approach to identifying the cause of disease and an Eastern approach to treating it. I like to know the exact physiological explanation behind diseases like cancer, heart disease, and arthritis. But when it comes to treating or preventing them, I rely on a holistic approach that includes herbs, diet, exercise, massage, rest, detoxification, positive thinking, meditation, and giving back.

The value of herbal formulas

If you walk into a store that sells herbal supplements you'll notice that the majority of products lining the shelves have just one herb. That's not necessarily because single-herb products work better than multi-herb products. It's just that they fit better with the Western way of thinking. Single-herb products are similar to pharmaceutical drugs in that both embrace the Western philosophy of disease treatment: one remedy for one condition. Of course, single herbs are much preferable to single drugs, because at least a whole herb often contains a variety of constituents that help balance each other, whereas a drug just contains one. But multi-herb formulas are even better when properly researched and formulated.

Both Traditional Chinese Medicine and Ayurveda rely on multi-herb formulas. In fact, you will never find a Traditional Chinese or Ayurvedic formula that has just one herb. That's because these millennia-old systems of healing recognize two important truths:

1. The whole is greater than the sum of its parts (meaning you'll get a greater effect from a blend of herbs than you will from just one).

2. Single substances usually have a therapeutic effect *and* a side effect. Therefore, each Eastern formula has a lead herb that is paired with secondary herbs that augment its actions and negate its side effects.

Based on these principles, I recommend the following herbal and nutrient combinations:

Lead ingredient: Cultured soy and curcumin
Secondary ingredients: Bioperine®, Ginger, Cardamom,
and Cinnamon

Cultured soy and curcumin go together very well. Each one falls under the category of "medicinal foods," meaning they are both foods and medicines. The traditional diets of China, Japan, Indonesia, and Singapore regularly incorporate small amounts of natural, cultured whole soy foods. Likewise, turmeric (which contains curcumin) has been used for centuries as a spice throughout India and Indonesia.

It turns out that the combination of these two botanical ingredients is more powerful than either ingredient alone. Research has shown that genistein, a key isoflavone in cultured soy, works synergistically with curcumin, meaning they enhance each other's anti-inflammatory and antioxidant effects.[111]

Have you ever wondered why we sprinkle pepper on our food? Our ancestors intuitively knew that pepper aids digestion and increases our body's ability to extract nutrients from food. For that reason, I like to pair curcumin with bioperine® (pronounced bio-PEAR-ine), a patented extract of black pepper. Research in animals and humans has shown that taking curcumin with bioperine dramatically increases its absorption.[112]

If you've ever eaten in an Indian restaurant you know it's very common to see ginger, cardamom, and cinnamon appear together. That specific combination has been used for centuries in Indian cooking. These herbs are the perfect complement to cultured soy, which is extremely effective as a nutritional supplement for people with terminal cancers and chronic infections. All three herbs have a strengthening effect on digestive health and immunity, both of which can be weakened in cancer patients.

Lead ingredient: Resveratrol
Secondary ingredients: Quercetin, Guggul, and Garlic

As you learned in Chapter Three, resveratrol has the remarkable ability to block age-related gene changes in the heart, in essence keeping it young. Quercetin (pronounced KWAIR-suh-ten) is a phyto-nutrient present in onions, broccoli, apples, and berries that appears to make resveratrol work better. How? Inside the human body, resveratrol can become chemically bound to other substances, limiting its ability to be absorbed. But when quercetin is thrown into the mix, it keeps resveratrol unbound, which could increase how much of it you absorb.[113, 114, 115]

Other ingredients I like to combine with resveratrol include guggul (pronounced GOO-gull) and garlic. Derived from the resin of an Indian tree, guggul is an Ayurvedic herb that has been shown to lower cholesterol and triglycerides. In fact, one human study found that taking guggul for three months caused a 24 percent drop in total cholesterol, and a 23 percent plunge in triglycerides in most patients.[116] Some animal research has shown that combining guggul with garlic produces even better results than guggul by itself.[117] Plus, garlic has its own heart benefits. Research has shown it lowers blood pressure, keeps blood cells from clumping together, prevents plaque formation in the arteries, and reduces cholesterol and triglyceride levels.[118]

Lead ingredient: Green tea
Secondary ingredients: B vitamins

A few years back, I was doing research on green tea with a team of researchers and a nutritionist. The research showed that green tea works synergistically with the B vitamins. In fact, both of them work in a similar way. Green tea boosts your metabolic rate, in other words, the rate at which you burn calories. B vitamins are essential for the production of energy, so they also aid your metabolism. The fact that green tea and B vitamins complement each other shouldn't be surprising, since vitamin B^{12} is actually found in tea leaves.

Interestingly, B vitamins also help manufacture the beneficial bacteria that reside in your digestive tract and which help keep the bad bacteria under control (Not all bacteria are bad as there are some strains that you actually *want* to have in your gut). That's an essential function, because if the bad bacteria take over they produce pro-inflammatory chemicals that, as we know, cause all kinds of trouble.

Unfortunately, good bacteria are easily destroyed by medications (particularly antibiotics), alcohol, smoking, an unhealthy diet, certain diseases and even stress. This means that most people in developed countries have far too many of the bad bacteria and far too few of the good. No wonder digestive difficulties are so rampant!

As you may recall, green tea is able to kill all sorts of microbes. So when you pair green tea with B vitamins, you're doing two complementary things – killing the bad bacteria, while promoting the growth of the good bacteria!

Lead ingredient: Ashwaghanda
Secondary ingredients: Shilajit, vitamin E

I really like the combination of ashwaghanda and shilajit (pronounced SHIL-i-jeet), which have both been used in Ayurveda for centuries. Shilajit is a mineral-rich rock sap. The same way that maple syrup can be extracted from maple trees, shilajit can be collected as it seeps out from certain mountains, such as the Himalayas.

Like ashwaghanda, shilajit belongs to a class of natural ingredients called adaptogens, so named because they help the body adapt to whatever condition it's facing. If you are tired or stressed out or worn thin, consider using these two herbs together because they make a great restorative combination.

In addition to acting as adaptogens, ashwaghanda and shilajit are often used in Ayurveda for their memory-improving and cognitive-enhancing effects in patients with dementia. Recent animal research shows there's some scientific validity to the ingredients' traditional use. Both ashwaghanda and shilajit appear to improve the brain's ability to use acetylcholine, a brain chemical that's essential to cognitive function.[119] Vitamin E is also a nice complement to ashwaghanda, as patients with Alzheimer's disease may have low levels of this antioxidant vitamin.[120]

Lead ingredient: Ginger
Secondary ingredients: Bromelain, Milk thistle, vitamin C

As we already discussed, ginger is an excellent herb for ailments of the digestive tract, including nausea, gas, abdominal pain, diarrhea, constipation, colic, and painful digestion. It may also be an effective treatment for inflammatory bowel disease. Ginger is wonderful when paired with bromelain, a group of digestive enzymes from pineapple. Each one works in a different way to alleviate indigestion. Ginger soothes painful stomach contractions, while bromelain helps break down foods, specifically protein.

In the West, we tend to think of digestion as taking place in the stomach. And certainly, the stomach plays a huge role in breaking down the foods we eat. But did you know that the liver is part of the digestive system too? If you want to support the whole system, it's best to take herbs that aid digestion, along with ones that support the proper functioning of the liver. And the best herb I know of for that purpose is milk thistle.

A traditional European herb, milk thistle has two main actions: it protects the liver from toxins and helps it recover from injury, including helping damaged parts of the liver grow back![121] In fact, most emergency rooms and poison control centers in Western Europe stock an extract of milk thistle because it is so effective in preventing liver damage and death from the accidental ingestion of death cap mushrooms.[122] Vitamin C also goes well with ginger and milk thistle because it acts as a catalyst that helps the body utilize other nutrients.

Lead ingredient: Lutein
Secondary ingredients: Zeaxanthin, Bilberry, Lycopene, vitamin A

Lutein, the yellow plant pigment that protects the macula of the eye from damaging UV rays, always occurs in nature with zeaxanthin (pronounced zee-uh-ZAN-thin). Interestingly, lutein and zeaxanthin are the only known plant pigments in the world that accumulate in the macula. So take a cue from nature. If you're going to take lutein, take it with zeaxanthin. They appear to work very closely together.

There are a number of other ingredients I recommend to people who want a complete approach to eye care. Lycopene, the antioxidant pigment that makes tomatoes red, is also found in eye tissue. Animal research indicates that lycopene protects against cataract development.[123] Bilberry, a relative of blueberry, relieves the effects of eyestrain and improves circulation to the eyes, which contain an intricate network of tiny blood vessels.[124] And vitamin A has long been recognized for its role in supporting healthy vision. People who have high blood levels of beta-carotene, the precursor of vitamin A are less likely to get cataracts or age-related macular degeneration than those with low levels.[125]

As you can see, when you use a combination of natural ingredients, you get more and better benefits that when you use just one. In the next chapter, you'll learn how natural ingredients can complement pharmaceutical drugs.

Chapter Five
How Natural Ingredients Complement Pharmaceutical Drugs

"Integrative medicine has much broader goals that simply giving doctors new tools. It aims to refocus medicine on health and healing rather than on disease and treatment, to restore the doctor-patient relationship that has so eroded in the present era of for-profit medicine, and to insist that human beings are more than physical bodies."[126]

-Dr. Andrew Weil (2004)

When it comes to alternative medicine people seem to be divided into two distinct camps. In one camp are those who believe that alternative therapies are little more than snake oil and that any benefits they produce are the result of a "placebo effect." In the other camp are those who think that alternative medicine is the answer to every health situation and that all pharmaceutical drugs are toxic. Fortunately, in the last decade, a third camp has emerged that embraces the middle ground. This camp is known as integrative medicine.

Integrative medicine acknowledges that there are some alternative therapies which are backed by scientific evidence of safety and efficacy, and some which are not. Likewise, it recognizes that while conventional medicine is excellent in some situations, while in others it is needlessly invasive and fraught with dangerous side effects. Accordingly, integrative medicine *integrates* the best therapies of both alternative and Western medicine. I am a proponent of integrative medicine. I believe both conventional and alternative therapies can play an important role in promoting optimal health.

In order to understand when to use Western medicine and when to use alternative medicine, it's important to identify the strengths of each. Western medicine is great for emergency situations. If you have a heart attack you don't want acupuncture – you want CPR. Conversely, alternative medicine is great at prevention. If your heart is healthy and you want to keep it that way, you don't need a pacemaker. You want to take resveratrol (in addition to eating a healthy diet and exercising!).

Alternative therapies are also helpful for treating long-term degenerative diseases such as Alzheimer's. While pharmaceutical drugs for Alzheimer's may slow down the progression of the disease, test tube and animal studies have shown that ashwaghanda may actually regenerate brain cells — something no drug has been able to do.

I also suggest using alternative medicine as a first line of treatment when tackling a problem that isn't life threatening. Why reach for the pharmaceutical drug Stemetil to quell nausea, which will have the side effect of destroying the beneficial bacteria in your gut, when you could take something safe and natural like ginger? If the ginger doesn't work you can always try the drug as a last resort.

Sometimes it's appropriate to use Western and alternative medicine at the same time. For example, chemotherapy and radiation will not work if a person is malnourished. Yet 25-50 percent of hospitalized cancer patients are malnourished![127] That's where cultured soy comes in. Research has shown it's extremely effective as a nutritional supplement for malnutrition, especially in people with terminal cancers. Another example is antibiotics. As effective as they are against bacteria, antibiotics aren't selective. In other words, they won't just kill the bad bacteria in your gut; they'll also kill the "good guys." So any time you take antibiotics, it's a good idea to take a potent B vitamin complex, because the B vitamins promote the growth of good bacteria. Not only that, recent test tube research indicates green tea actually boosts antibiotics' ability to kill disease-causing bacteria![128]

Probiotics (supplements of live, beneficial bacteria) are also a good complement to antibiotics. A final example is statin drugs. These prescription medications are excellent at lowering cholesterol, but they also lower levels of coenzyme Q_{10}, a nutrient that's necessary for cellular health. Therefore, you always want to take statin drugs in combination with CoQ_{10} supplements. Whatever route you decide to pursue – alternative, Western, or integrative medicine, – always consult with a qualified health care practitioner to help you plan your health regimen.

Drug discovery from natural sources
There are 121 prescription drugs in use Today which come from 90 plant species. About 74% came from the following folklore claims.
(Benowitz, S., The Scientist 10, 1996, 1-7)

>Approximately 25% of the drug prescriptions in the USA are compounds derived from plants and were discovered through scientific investigation of folklore claims.
(Reynold, T., Nat'l Cancer Inst, 183, 1991, 594-596)

**Why are natural products
A good source of anticancer drugs?**

Almost 74% (48/65) of all drugs approved either were natural products, were based thereon or mimicked them in one form or another (1981-2002)

*Newman, DJ, Cragg GM, Snader KM,
J. Nat. Prod, 2003, 66, 1022-1037*

Chapter Six
Living Inflammation-Free

"As individuals, we hold our futures in the palms of our hands. We can choose to ignore the evidence and take our chances with long-term health. Or we can take many steps to improve our chances of having a long and healthy life."
-Jack Challem, author of The Inflammation Syndrome (2003)

Every day, you make a dozen or more choices that affect the levels of inflammation in your body. What you eat, how often you exercise, how much you sleep, your level of exposure to toxic chemicals inside and outside the home ... even the feelings you experience can all impact whether your body produces more anti-inflammatory chemicals or pro-inflammatory ones.

My goal is to move you out of a chronic state of inflammation and toward a state of health. To that end, taking the herbs featured in this book is a great starting place. But, those herbs will be even more effective if you make conscious lifestyle choices too. Since all of the conditions in this book share a common thread of inflammation, the lifestyle recommendations for one disease are the same as for the others.

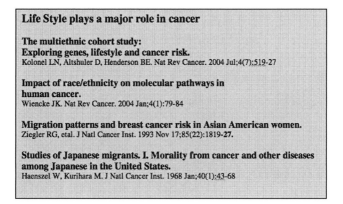

Life Style plays a major role in cancer

The multiethnic cohort study:
Exploring genes, lifestyle and cancer risk.
Kolonel LN, Altshuler D, Henderson BE. Nat Rev Cancer. 2004 Jul;4(7):519-27

Impact of race/ethnicity on molecular pathways in human cancer.
Wiencke JK. Nat Rev Cancer. 2004 Jan;4(1):79-84

Migration patterns and breast cancer risk in Asian American women.
Ziegler RG, etal. J Natl Cancer Inst. 1993 Nov 17;85(22):1819-27.

Studies of Japanese migrants. I. Morality from cancer and other diseases among Japanese in the United States.
Haenszel W, Kurihara M. J Natl Cancer Inst. 1968 Jan;40(1):43-68

Eat smart

One of the most powerful tools at your disposal to fight inflammation is your diet. That's great news, because unlike factors such as outdoor air quality, which you can't individually do much about, what you eat is totally within your control. Each time you sit down to a meal, you can make food choices that either raise or lower the level of inflammation in your body.

It probably won't surprise you to learn which foods promote inflammation, because they're the same foods you already know are bad for you: white flour products and other refined grains (white bread, rice, pasta, and crackers), trans fats (any food that has been deep-fried or contains the word "hydrogenated" in the list of ingredients), sugary foods (fruit is okay, but steer clear of cookies, donuts, cakes, and sodas), and meats high in saturated fat (bacon, sausage, salami, etc.). Even vegetable oils (corn, safflower, sunflower, and soybean oils), which many experts have touted as healthy, are actually pro-inflammatory. As you may have noticed, the typical Western diet is heavy on foods that promote inflammation!

When levels of inflammation are high, you are more likely to develop a resistance to insulin, the hormone that keeps your blood sugar levels balanced. That's why eating pro-inflammatory foods increase your risk for diabetes (in addition to the diseases we've already covered in this book). Fortunately, about 80 percent of our ability to lower insulin levels rests with our dietary choices.

So what should you eat? Take a page from the people of the Mediterranean region (Crete, Greece, and southern Italy), who have followed a naturally anti-inflammatory diet for centuries. Research has shown that people who eat a traditional Mediterranean diet are less likely to die of *all causes* discussed in this book than those who follow a modern Western diet.[129]

1. Eat lots of fruits and vegetables. Study after study has shown that fruits and veggies (which contain impressive stores of anti-inflammatory and antioxidant phyto-nutrients), protect against many different diseases, including heart disease, cancer, and arthritis.

2. Include at least two to three servings per week of cold-water fatty fish, such as salmon, tuna, mackerel, herring, anchovy, trout, and sardines. These fish are rich in anti-inflammatory omega-3 fatty acids.

3. Use olive oil as your primary cooking oil. Unlike other fats, olive oil lowers total cholesterol and LDL (bad) cholesterol.

4. Emphasize whole grain products, beans, nuts, and seeds. Foods in their whole state have more fiber, vitamins, and phyto-nutrients than refined and processed foods.

5. Eat only lean meats from free-range or grass-fed animals, which

contain higher amounts of good fats and lower amounts of bad fats than factory-farmed and corn-fed animals.

Get moving

If you're like 60 percent of Americans, you don't exercise regularly.[130] It's not something to be ashamed of. It can be difficult to make time to exercise with today's busy schedules. However, I encourage you to get moving in whatever way you can, because exercise is one of the best things you can do for your health.

There are so many reasons why exercising is good for you. It improves your heart function, tones your muscles, increases your lung capacity, and benefits your mood. But, new research also shows that exercise reduces the amount of inflammation in your body. A number of studies comparing athletes to couch potatoes have found that people who exercise regularly have lower blood levels of CRP (the indicator of body-wide inflammation) than people who are inactive.[131] The good news is that you can reverse this situation immediately. When inactive people get off the couch and start exercising, their CRP levels go down within weeks.[132]

Most people think of exercise as anything that makes you sweat, but a balanced exercise program will include three elements:

1. Aerobic exercise (activities that get your heart rate up, such as jogging, biking, sports, aerobics, dancing, etc.),

2. Strength training (lifting weights), and

3. Stretching (either on your own or in a yoga class). Ideally, you want to exercise aerobically six days a week, do strength training three days a week, and stretch on the other four days. Stretching won't help you lose fat or build muscle, but it will help to prevent the injuries that can keep you from exercising.

Don't feel like you have to become an athlete overnight (or ever!). Do what's comfortable for you. Even a small amount of activity can have a big impact. For example, taking a brisk, thirty-minute walk three days a week can lower your blood pressure and improve your overall fitness.[133]

Also, keep in mind that getting fit doesn't mean losing weight. You can be thin and unhealthy, and you can be overweight and healthy. Some people, especially women, may spend an extraordinary amount of hours in the gym and have very little externally to show for their efforts. Why? Because exercise burns dangerous visceral fat (the kind that collects around the belly and organs). But, it has a much smaller impact on subcutaneous fat (the kind that collects on the hips, thighs, and buttocks). That's why women have a harder time losing fat than men. Men tend to accumulate easy-to-lose belly fat, while women tend to accumulate hard-to-lose subcutaneous fat.

Get regular massages

While some people might consider massages an indulgence, I prefer to look at them as part of an exercise program. Exercising keeps everything flowing in your body – your blood, your lymphatic fluids, even what Chinese health practitioners call "chi" (pronounced "chee") or vital life energy. Massage has similar benefits. It's wonderful for getting rid of knots and tension, but it also increases blood and lymphatic circulation. Additionally, a good massage will help move toxins out of the areas where they usually congregate (the buttocks, belly, and back muscles) and promote their excretion. So you want to get that regular massage, whether it's every week, every two weeks, or every three weeks.

There are many different kinds of massage techniques including shiatsu (a Japanese pressure point therapy), rolfing (a soft-tissue manipulation technique designed to realign the body), Swedish (which uses long, flowing strokes), and Ayurvedic (an oil massage performed with two therapists, one working on either side of the body). Experiment and find the one that's right for you.

Give yourself the gift of sleep

Sleep is underrated. When life gets hectic, sleep is usually the first thing to go, because we know we can "get by" on fewer hours than our bodies would like. But just because we may be able to function in the face of chronic sleep deprivation doesn't mean it doesn't have consequences. Research shows that getting less than six or seven hours of sleep a night increases your risk of all kinds of diseases, including cancer, heart disease, diabetes, and obesity.[134]

Scientists suspect that when you wake up before your natural sleep cycle is complete, your body assumes there must be a life-threatening reason. Why else would you deprive yourself of this necessity? The response is to produce stress hormones and increase blood pressure so you can manage the "threat." Your immune system also kicks into high gear, releasing inflammatory chemicals into the bloodstream to prepare for a possible injury. Interestingly, just *one night* of inadequate sleep can cause your levels of inflammation to rise.[135] Imagine what chronic sleep deprivation does!

Give yourself the gift of sleep. Skimp on other things like television, catching up on the news, or surfing the Internet, before you skimp on sleep. Your body will appreciate it!

Detoxify your home

When you think of toxic places, you probably imagine hazardous waste sites or cities that have been the victim of nuclear accidents, such as Chernobyl. But did you know that your home may contain unsafe levels of toxins too?

According to studies conducted by the Environmental Protection Agency, the air inside the average home is two to five times more polluted than the air right outside its walls.[136] Why? Because everyday items we think of as benign are actually quite toxic. Paint, particle board (used to make furniture in place of real wood), carpeting, upholstery, and freshly dry cleaned clothing all emit volatile organic compounds (VOCs), which are toxic chemicals that trigger inflammation in the body. You may also be exposed to VOCs if you use synthetic household cleansers and disinfectants, air fresheners, perfumes, and pesticides. Some simple steps will reduce your exposure to these toxins and protect you from inflammation.

The easiest measure you can take to detoxify your home is to switch from chemically laden products to natural brands. Swap your regular household cleansers for non-toxic alternatives, your chemical air fresheners for plant-derived essential oils, and your synthetic perfumes for botanical ones. Search for a chemically-free dry cleaner or let your freshly dry chemically cleaned clothes outgas (emit all their VOCs) outside for a couple days before bringing them in. Inside the home use roach and ant traps instead of chemical sprays and, outside the home, forgo the toxic garden chemicals and choose natural fertilizers and weed killers instead. And always open the doors and windows when using paint, paint strippers or other solvents, glues, and even hairspray.

You may also want to invest in products that make your home a healthier place. For example, a good water filter will protect you from the contaminants in your tap water (not the least of which is chlorine). A quality air filter will help reduce levels of indoor air pollution. And full-spectrum light bulbs, which emulate the full spectrum of colors and wavelengths found in sunlight, may improve your mood, reduce your stress levels, and increase your productivity.

If you're really committed to detoxifying your home, you can also take more involved steps. Choose low-VOC paint for the inside of your home. Go for natural fabrics such as wool over synthetic when buying carpeting and upholstered furniture. Replace your mattress that is probably doused with flame retardant chemicals with an organic mattress that is free of these toxins. And buy real wood furniture over pieces made with particle board (Or if that's too expensive, buy used furniture, which has already given off all its VOCs). In other words, whenever you have a choice between products that will fill the air with chemicals and those that won't, choose the ones that won't!

Detoxify your body

Considering the amount of toxins we encounter every day — in our homes, at our workplaces, in the food we eat, the water we drink, and the air we breathe — it's a good idea to detoxify your body every six months too. Otherwise, you will store these toxic chemicals in your fatty tissues where they can stay for decades, contributing to inflammation and ultimately harming your health. According to a study conducted at the Mt. Sinai School of Medicine in New York, the average person has traces of ninety-one toxic chemicals in the blood and urine.[137]

There are two ways you can go about cleansing. If you can afford it, I recommend signing up for a detoxification program at a health and wellness center. At the Hippocrates Health Institute in West Palm Beach, Florida, for example, you can experience detoxifying treatments such as colon hydrotherapy, where the colon is gently irrigated with water to remove toxic waste build-up from the intestines; cellulite massage that is designed to rid your body of toxins that manifest as cellulite deposits; and reflexology, which helps the body release toxins by activating points on the feet associated with different organs.

My personal favorite detoxification program is panchakarma therapy, which you can find at Maharishi Ayurveda Centers around the country. Literally meaning "five actions," panchakarma is a complex detoxification program that includes procedures which may seem strange to Westerners, but which have been used successfully in India for centuries. These include oil massage, sweat therapy, nasal massage, purging, herbal enemas, and blood purification. A recent study found that panchakarma reduced levels of certain fat-soluble toxins by 50 percent after five days of treatment.[138]

Alternatively, you can work with a qualified health care practitioner in your area. He or she will access your level of wellness and recommend some gentle detox programs you can do at home, which will likely include a cleansing diet and detoxifying herbs. Sometimes the practitioner may recommend colon hydrotherapy; however, if you opt for colonics, I would strongly urge you to be under the supervision of a naturopathic or holistic physician.

There is no one correct right way to detoxify. Choose what is comfortable for you. Just don't go it alone!

Change your mind

Whether you view the glass as half empty or half full has a profound impact on your health. Optimists are 23 percent less likely to die of heart failure than pessimists — and a whopping 55 percent less likely to die from causes such as those discussed in this book.[139] In a prime example of the mind-body connection, negative feelings such as depression, anxiety, hostility, and stress can cause your body to release a slew of inflammatory chemicals that put you at risk for disease.[140]

While we may seem like slaves to our emotions, we have more control over them than we believe. Certainly there are people who suffer from chronic depression or anxiety that need professional guidance. But many times, the simple process of examining our thoughts can set us free from them.

When we take time to notice the thoughts that are causing us to feel a certain way, we get a little distance from them. We can question whether the thoughts are really true, instead of blindly accepting and reacting to them. For example, if the thought "No one appreciates how hard I work" passes through your head, instead of believing it and feeling depressed or angry, ask yourself "Is that really true? Is it true that not one person in the entire world appreciates how hard I work?" Most of the time, you'll find these destructive thoughts aren't actually true, and only serve to harm your emotional and physical health

Here is a simple, scientifically tested way to boost your happiness and maybe extend your life. Every evening before you go to bed, take five minutes to jot down three things about your day that went well and why. Research shows that doing this easy little exercise for just a week boosts happiness levels for an amazing *six months*.[141] There's a reason the words "gratitude" and "gratification" are so closely related in the English language: Gratitude leads to gratification.

Meditate

When I recommend to people is that they start a daily meditation practice, a lot of them tell me they don't know how to meditate. The truth is, meditation is very simple. It's essentially just sitting quietly and reconnecting with the wisdom of your body. When you sit in silence, and turn your attention away from your thoughts and toward your body, you learn how to listen to what it's telling you. You may notice tension in your neck and shoulders. You may notice your heartbeat is anxious or erratic. You may notice your breathing is shallow. All of these are important messages from your body, telling you to stretch, or to do something relaxing, or to breathe deeply. But unless you sit quietly in attention, you won't get the messages!

I find that if people are leading a typically busy life but are not meditating, they are not in touch with the wisdom of their bodies. The moment you can quietly observe that you're feeling anxious or moody or stressed is the moment that emotion stops ruling you. When you listen to your body, you know the action you need to employ to take care of yourself. Your body always has the answers if you are willing to listen.

There are many types of meditation to choose from, including guided imagery (listening to a tape that guides you to visualize something relaxing), transcendental meditation (a method that uses personal mantra recitation), vipassana (an ancient form that focuses on noticing physical sensations of the body), and mindfulness meditation (which trains attention away from the thoughts and toward the breath). You can choose what feels right to you. You can meditate at home or in classes. You can even attend silent meditation retreats. The important thing is consistency: It's better to meditate for ten minutes every day than for an hour once a week.

Give back

According to happiness researcher Dr. Martin Seligman, one of the keys to happiness is serving something larger than yourself.[142] And, as we've already established, happy people have lower levels of inflammation! So pick something that is personally meaningful to you, whether that is a big cause like the fight against cancer, or something that's closer to home, like your local animal shelter. Then volunteer a little of your time (even if it's just one hour a month) anything that gives back and serves. There is tremendous peace and satisfaction that can be gained from transcending the small details of your life in order to make the world a better place.

My way of giving back is to take part in an international non-governmental organization called READ that is near and dear to the heart of my partner, former California Senator and international humanist, Omer Rains, who serves on its International Board of Directors. READ (an acronym for "Rural Education and Development") builds libraries and economic development centers in rural and remote parts of the developing world. So far, this tireless and devoted organization has built close to fifty (50) libraries throughout Nepal and India, and has plans to expand its program into five more countries in the developing world over the next three years. It feels so good to know that I am making a difference by contributing to and participating with an organization such as READ!

PREVENT CANCER

Conclusion

Many people hold a mistaken belief that whether we retain our health or succumb to disease is all in our genes. They don't realize that the everyday choices we make have an incredible amount of power to change the course of our lives. Just because you have a strong family history of a certain disease doesn't consign you to a doomsday scenario. I am a living example of this fact. I have a family history of diabetes — my father, both of my grandmothers, and several of my aunts are diabetics. About two years ago, I too was diagnosed with diabetes. I didn't take the diagnosis lightly, considering it's the seventh leading cause of death in the United States. Through dietary changes and nutritional supplements, however, I completely reversed the condition. To this day, my physician is baffled.

It is my hope that this book has made a compelling case for the importance of fighting body-wide inflammation, and given you the tools to do so. I have seen the destructive effects of inflammation on my life, the lives of my patients and the people I love. I have also witnessed the power that lifestyle changes and natural anti-inflammatory remedies can have in bringing people back to a state of health and wellness. May this information help you and your loved ones lead a long and healthy life.

PREVENT CANCER

Resource Directory
Natural Health Care Modalities and Recommended Resources

Ayurvedic Medicine
•Ayurvedic Health Center Online
www.ayurvedic.org
•American Academy of Ayurvedic Medicine
Ph: (732) 247-3301
www.ayurvedicacademy.com
•Maharishi Ayurvedic Center
www.tm.org

Biofeedback
•Biofeedback Certification Institute of America
Ph (303) 420-2902
www.bcia.org

Chinese Herbs
•Acupuncture.com: The Online Resource for Traditional Medicine
www.acupuncture.com

Chiropractic
•American Chiropractic Association
Ph (703) 276-8800
www.amerchiro.org

Craniosacral Therapy
•The Upledger Institute, Inc
Ph: (800) 233-5880
www.upledger.com

Flower Remedies
•Flower Essence Society
www.flowersociety.org

Guided Imagery
•The Academy for Guided Imagery
Ph: (800) 726-2070
Website: www.healthy.net/agi

Energy Medicine
•Emotional Freedom Technique by Gary Craig
www.emotionalfreedomtechnique.com
•Reconnection Energy
www.thereconnection.com

Reiki
•International Center for Reiki Training
Ph: (800) 332 8112
www.reiki.org
•QiGong Database
The Qi Gong Institute
Ph: (415) 323 1221
www.healthy.net/qigonginstitute

Herbal Medicine
•American Botanical Council
Ph: (512) 926-4900
www.herbalgram.org
•Herb Research Foundation
Ph: (300) 449-2265
www.herbs.org

Holistic Dentistry
•Holistic Dental Association
www.holisticdental.org

Holistic Medicine
•American Holistic Medical Association (AHMA)
www.ahmaholistic.com
•American College for Advancement in Medicine (ACAM)
Ph: (800) 532-3688
•American Association of Naturopathic Physicians (AANP)
www.naturopathic.org
•Foundation for the Advancement of Innovative Medicine (FAIM)
E-mail: faim@rockland.net

Homeopathy
•Homeopathic Academy of Naturopathic Physicians
Ph: (503) 761-3298
http://www.hanp.net/
•National Center for Homeopathy
Ph: (703) 548-7790
www.homeopathic.org

Massage Therapy
•American Massage Therapy Association
www.inet.amtammasge.org
•Touch Research Institute
www.miami.edu/touch-research

Naturopathic Medicine
•American Association of Naturopathic Physicians
Ph: (866) -538-2267
www.naturopathic.org

Osteopathic Medicine
•American Osteopathic Association
Ph: (800) 621-1773
www.aoa-net.org

Polarity Therapy
•American Polarity Therapy Association (APTA)
www.polaritytherapy.org

Reflexology
•Home of Reflexology
www.reflexology.org
•Reflexology Research
www.reflexology-research.com

Relaxation Response
•The Mind/Body Medical Institute
www.med.harvard.edu/programs/mindbody

Therapeutic Touch
•American Holistic Nurses' Association
www.ahma.org
•Healing Touch International
www.healingtouch.net

Traditional Chinese Medicine
•American Association of Oriental Medicine
Ph: (610) 266-1433
www.aaom.org
•Acupuncure.com: The OnlineResource for
Traditional Chinese Medicine
www.acupuncture.com

Transcendental Meditation
•The Transcendental Meditation Program
www.tm.org

Yoga
•American Yoga Association
Ph: (941) 927-4977
•Yoga Journal
www.yogajournal.com
•Yoga Research Center
http://yogaresearchcenter.com/

Resources for Recommended Dietary Supplements
•JIVA—Essence of Life
487 East Main Street, Suite 297
Mt. Kisco, NY 10549
Ph (800) 517-7606
www.jivasupplements.org
•Long Life Catalog
Natural Supplements
PO Box 36
E. Canaan, CT 06024
888-217-7233
www.longlifecatalogs.com

•Life Extension Foundation.
www.lifeextensionfoundation.com
•Arjuna Himalaya USA
www.himalayausa.com
•Total Health Discount Vitamins
120 Broadhollow Road, Suite 1
Farmingdale, NY 11735
Ph (800)- 283-2833
www.totaldiscountvitamins.com

General Sites about Alternative Medicine
•The Alternative Medicine Home Page
www.pitt.edu/-chw/altm.html
•American Holistic Health Association (AHHA)
www.ahha.org
•Dr. Andrew Weil
www.drweil.com
•HealthAtoZ
www.healthatoz.com
•Prevention's Healthy Ideas™
www.healthyideas.com
•Journey to Wellness
www.journeytowellnessnow.com
•Wellness Web
www.wellweb.com

PREVENT CANCER

Glossary

anti-nutrient: a substance that prevents the body from absorbing nutrients, such as essential minerals and trace elements

antioxidant: a substance that protects the cells from the damaging effects of oxidants

ashwaganda: an ancient Ayurvedic herb that helps the body adapt to stress and may improve brain function in cases of dementia (including Alzheimer's)

Ayurveda: the ancient medical system of India

B vitamins: key nutrients essential for the production of energy and the manufacture of beneficial bacteria

bilberry: a relative of the blueberry that relieves the effects of eye strain and improves circulation to the eyes

bioperine: a patented extract of black pepper that dramatically increases the absorption of curcumin

bromelain: a group of digestive enzymes from pineapple

C-reactive protein (CRP): an indicator of chronic body-wide inflammation

coenzyme Q_{10}: a nutrient necessary for cellular health that is depleted with the use of statin drugs

cultured soy: a nutritious, easily digestible and almost hypoallergenic type of soy that is used in the prevention and treatment of cancer

culturing: the process of adding beneficial microbial cultures to a food and letting them transform it into something more nutritious and digestible

curcumin: the major constituent of turmeric, an herb used for thousands of years to treat a variety of inflammatory diseases

daidzein: a phyto-nutrient found in soy that has been shown to work with genistein to fight cancer in multiple ways

dementia: the loss of thinking ability that happens when brain cells die

ECGC: a phyto-nutrient in green tea with powerful antioxidant activity

free radical: a substance that steals an electron from another molecule through a reaction with oxygen (also "oxidant")

garlic: a spicy herb that works in multiple ways to protect cardiovascular health

genistein: a phyto-nutrient found in soy that has been shown to work with daidzein to fight cancer in multiple ways

ginger: a spicy herb that has been used in some of the world's major herbal traditions to treat ailments of the digestive tract

green tea: lightly steamed leaves of the *Camellia sinensis* shrub (the same plant from which black tea is derived), which provide sustained energy without the crash of stimulants

guggul: an Ayurvedic herb derived from the resin of an Indian tree and shown to lower cholesterol and triglycerides

Heliobacter pylori: the bacterium that causes ulcers

HDL cholesterol: high density lipoprotein, or "good" cholesterol

inflammation: a response of the immune system — which includes redness, heat, pain and swelling — to a real or perceived threat that, when chronic, contributes to many serious diseases

integrative medicine: a system of medicine that incorporates the best therapies of both alternative and Western medicine

LDL cholesterol: low density lipoprotein, or "bad" cholesterol

lutein: a yellow pigment found in plants that accumulates in the macula of the eye, where it protects that structure from damaging UV rays

macula: the part of the eye located at the back of the retina that is responsible for sharp central vision

macular degeneration: a serious eye disease that slowly destroys central vision

milk thistle: a traditional European herb that protects the liver from toxins and helps it recover from injury

nuclear factor kappa-B (NF-kB): a protein that plays a key role in initiating inflammation by turning certain genes on or off

oxidant: a substance that steals an electron from another molecule through a reaction with oxygen (also "free radical")

oxidized cholesterol: cholesterol that has been attacked — and therefore damaged — by free radicals

phyto-nutrient: a beneficial compound found in plants

plaques and tangles: two abnormal, nerve-killing structures that develop in the brains of Alzheimer's patients

probiotics: supplements of live, beneficial bacteria

quercetin: a phyto-nutrient present in onions, broccoli, apples and berries that appears to make resveratrol work better

resveratrol: a phyto-nutrient found in the skin of red grapes and wine that blocks age-related gene changes in the heart

shilajit: a mineral-rich rock sap that has been used in Ayurveda for centuries to help the body adapt to stress and improve memory and cognition

synovial joint: a joint in which the two bones meeting are bathed in synovia, a clear fluid whose job is to provide lubrication

Traditional Chinese Medicine: the ancient medical system of China

vitamin A: an essential nutrient that has long been recognized for its role in supporting healthy vision

vitamin C: an essential nutrient and antioxidant that acts as a catalyst to help the body utilize other nutrients

vitamin E: an essential nutrient and antioxidant that may be deficient in people with Alzheimer's

zeaxanthin: a sister pigment to lutein that also provides protection to the macula of the eye from UV damage

References (Endnotes)

1 Leaf, Clifton. "Why we're losing the war on cancer (and how to win it)." *Fortune*. Vol. 149, No.6. March 22, 2004.

2 Aggarwal, Bharat B. "Natural products for forging east-west relationships and working together to create new medicines." CHI's 14th Annual Molecular Medicine Tri-Conference, Clinical Trials in India & Asia: Feb. 27-March 2, 2007. Moscone North Convention Center, San Francisco, CA.

3 Gorman, Christine; Park, Alice; Dell, Kristina. "The fires within." *Time*. Feb 23, 2004.

4 Rowland, Rhonda. "Inflammation appears to do a number on human heart." *CNN*. Nov. 13, 2000. http://archives.cnn.com/2000/HEALTH/11/13/heart.inflammation/ (Accessed July 30, 2008.)

5 Meggs, William Joel; Svec, Carol. *The Inflammation Cure*. McGraw-Hill: New York, 2004, p. 51.

6 Meggs, p. 54.

7 Wheeler, Mark. "UCLA researchers identify the molecular signature of loneliness." *UCLA Newsroom*. Sept. 13, 2007. http://newsroom.ucla.edu/portal/ucla/Loneliness-Is-a-Molecule-UCLA-8214.aspx?RelNum=8214 (Accessed July 30, 2008.)

8 Meggs, p. 87.

9 Centers for Disease Control. "Arthritis and chronic joint symptoms more common than previously thought." *United States Department of Health and Human Services, Centers for Disease Control and Prevention*. Oct. 24, 2002. http://www.cdc.gov/od/oc/media/pressrel/r021024.htm (Accessed July 30, 2008.)

10 University of Washington Medicine. "Aspirin and related drugs (NSAIDS)." *University of Washington Medicine*. May 11, 2007. http://www.orthop.washington.edu/uw/medications/tabID__3376/ItemID__72/PageID__34/Articles/Default.aspx (Accessed July 30, 2008.)

11 Drugs.com. "Ibuprofen." Drugs.com. Revised March 26, 2008. http://www.drugs.com/ibuprofen.html (Accessed July 30, 2008.)

12 Lee, Daniel. "Tylenol (Acetaminophen) causes liver damage." MedicineNet.com. Last editorial review Aug. 27, 2007. http://www.medicinenet.com/tylenol_liver_damage/article.htm (Accessed July 30, 2008.)

13 Bombardier C, et al. Comparison of upper gastrointestinal toxicity of rofecoxib and naproxen in patients with rheumatoid arthritis. VIGOR Study Group. *N Engl J Med*. 2001 May 3;344(18):1398.

14 Siegfried, Donna Rae. "First Vioxx, then Bextra, now Celebrex?" *Arthritis Today*. Feb 28, 2005.

15 CNNMoney.com. "Pfizer cites Celebrex heart attack risk." *CNNMoney*.

com. Dec. 17, 2004. http://money.cnn.com/2004/12/17/news/fortune500/
pfizer/index.htm (Accessed July 30, 2008.)

16 American Heart Association. "Inflammation, heart disease and stroke:
The role of C-reactive protein." *American Heart Association.* http://www.
americanheart.org/presenter.jhtml?identifier=4648 (Accessed July 30, 2008.)

17 Gorman, 2004.

18 American Heart Association.

19 Gorman, 2004.

20 Consumer Health Information Network. "Corticosteroids." *Consumer
Health Information Network.* July 9, 2008. http://arthritis-symptom.com/
arthritis-drugs/corticosteroids.htm (Accessed July 30, 2008.)

21 Azer, Samy. "Colitis." *eMedicine Health.* Last editorial review Oct. 4,
2005. http://www.emedicinehealth.com/colitis/article_em.htm (Accessed July
31, 2008.)

22 National Digestive Diseases Information Clearinghouse. "Crohn's disease." *National Digestive Diseases Information Clearinghouse, a service
of the National Institute of Diabetes and Digestive and Kidney Diseases,
National Institutes of Health.* Feb. 2006. http://digestive.niddk.nih.gov/ddis-
eases/pubs/crohns/index.htm (Accessed July 31, 2008.)

23 Russel M. Changes in the incidence of inflammatory bowel disease: what
does it mean? *Eur J Intern Med.* 2000 Aug;11(4):191-196.

24 Pons, Mauricio E, Garcia-Valenzuela, Enrique. "Macular degeneration."
eMedicine Health. Last editorial review April 20, 2007. http://www.emedi-
cinehealth.com/macular_degeneration/article_em.htm (Accessed July 31,
2008.)

25 University of Utah Health Sciences Center. "New gene linked to macular
degeneration risk." *ScienceDaily* Oct. 19, 2006. http://www.sciencedaily.com
/releases/2006/10/061019192829.htm
(Accessed July 31, 2008.)

26 University of Illinois Eye & Ear Infirmary. "Macular degeneration info."
The Eye Digest. Reviewed 17 June 2007. http://www.agingeye.net/macularde-
gen/maculardegeninformation.php (Accessed July 31, 2008.)

27 University of Illinois Eye & Ear Infirmary, 2007.

28 Schmidt R, et al. Early inflammation and dementia: a 25-year follow-up
of the Honolulu-Asia Aging Study. *Ann Neurol.* 2002 Aug;52(2):168-74.

29 Meggs, p. 94.

30 Breggin, Peter. *The Anti-Depressant Fact Book: What Your Doctor Won't
Tell You About Prozac, Zoloft, Paxil, Celexa and Luvox.* Perseus Publishing:
Cambridge, MA, 2001, p. 137.

31 Nelson, Nathan C. "The free radical theory of aging." *Department of
Physics, Ohio State University.* http://www.physics.ohio-state.edu/~wilkins/

writing/Samples/shortmed/nelson/radicals.html (Accessed July 31, 2008.)

32 Better Health Channel. "Antioxidants." *State of Victoria (Australia).* Nov. 2007. http://www.betterhealth.vic.gov.au/bhcv2/bhcarticles.nsf/pages/ Antioxidants?open (Accessed July 31, 2008.)

33 Knight JA. Review: Free radicals, antioxidants, and the immune system. *Annals Clin Lab Sci.* 2000;30(2):145-158.

34 Gorman, 2004.

35 Stapans I, et al. Oxidized cholesterol in the diet accelerates the development of atherosclerosis in LDL receptor- and apolipoprotein E-deficient mice. *Arterioscler Thromb Vasc Biol.* 2000;20:708.

36 Colebank, Susan. "Deconstructing soy." *Health Supplement Retailer.* April 2, 2002. http://www.naturalproductsmarketplace.com/ articles/241feat1.html (Accessed Aug. 15, 2008)

37 Fallon, Sally. "The ploy of soy." *Nourished Magazine.* http://editor.nourishedmagazine.com.au/articles/the-ploy-of-soy (Accessed Aug. 15, 2008)

38 University of Illinois at Urbana-Champaign (2008, March 9). "Can allergic reactions to soy be overcome through fermentation?" *ScienceDaily.* http://www.sciencedaily.com /releases/2008/03/080306113750.htm (Accessed Aug. 18, 2008)

39 Anderson, Nina in cooperation with Dr. Howard Peiper. *Cancer Disarmed: Healing Benefits of a Fermented and Nitrogenated Soy.* Safe Goods Publishing: Sheffield, MA, 2004, p.24.

40 Messina MJ, et al. Soy intake and cancer risk: a review of the in vitro and in vivo data. *Nutr. Cancer.* 1994;21(2):113-31.

41 Wu AH, et al. Adolescent and adult soy intake and risk of breast cancer in Asian-Americans. *Carcinogenesis.* Sep;23(9):1491-6.

42 Nagata Y, et al. Dietary isoflavones may protect against prostate cancer in Japanese men. *J Nutr.* 2007 Aug;13(8):1974-9.

43 A clinical study of Haelen 851 concentrated nutritional oral liquid in supporting healthy energy and lowering toxic effects of radiation and chemotherapy on cancer patients. *U.S. Research Reports, Inc.* April 1, 1993.

44 Khopde SM, et al. Free radical scavenging ability and antioxidant efficiency of curcumin and its substituted analogue. *Biophys Chem.* 1999;80:85-91.

45 Mukhopadhyay A, et al. Anti-inflammatory and irritant activities of curcumin analogues in rats. *Agents Actions.* 1982;12:508-515.

46 Shishodia S, Sethi G, Aggarwal B. Curcumin: Getting back to the roots. *Ann NY Acad Sci.* 2005 Nov;1056:206-17.

47 Joe B, et al. Presence of an acidic glycoprotein in the serum of arthritic rats: modulation by capsaicin and curcumin. *Mol Cell Biochem.* 1997 Apr;169(1-2):125-34.

48 Funk JL, et al. Efficacy and mechanism of action of turmeric

supplements in the treatment of experimental arthritis. *Arthritis Rheum.* 2006 Nov;54(11):3452-64.

49 Innes JF, et al. Randomised, double-blind, placebo-controlled parallel group study of P54FP for the treatment of dogs with osteoarthritis. *Vet Rec.* 2003 Apr 12;152(15):457-60.

50 McCaleb, R., Leigh, E. and K. Morien. *The Encyclopedia of Popular Herbs. Your Complete Guide to the Leading Medicinal Plants.* Roseville, CA: Prima Health, 2000, pp. 378.

51 Shakibaei M, et al. Suppression of NF-kappaB activation by curcumin leads to inhibition of expression of cyclo-oxygenase-2 and matrix metallo-proteinase-9 in human articular chondrocytes: Implications for the treatment of osteoarthritis. *Biochem Pharmacol.* 2007 May 1;73(9):1434-45.

52 Park C, et al. Curcumin induces apoptosis and inhibits prostaglandin E(2) production in synovial fibroblasts of patients with rheumatoid arthritis. *Int J Mol Med.* 2007 Sep;20(3):365-72.

53 Baur JA, et al. Resveratrol improves health and survival of mice on a high-calorie diet. *Nature.* 2006 Nov 16;444(7117):337-42.

54 Barger JL. A low dose of dietary resveratrol partially mimics calorie restriction and retards aging parameters in mice. *PLoS ONE.* 2008. 3(6): e2264. doi:10.1371/journal.pone.0002264. (Accessed Aug. 24, 2008)

55 Editorial. "Of red wine and fatty foods." *The New York Times.* Nov. 3, 2006. http://www.nytimes.com/2006/11/03/opinion/03fri3.html (Accessed Aug. 24, 2008)

56 Seligman, Katherine. "Can a diet of a quarter fewer calories than a body needs lead Boomers to that ever elusive fountain of youth?" *San Francisco Gate.* Sept. 2, 2007. http://www.sfgate.com/cgi-bin/article.cgi?f=/c/a/2007/09/02/CM0CRASBE.DTL (Accessed Aug. 24, 2008)

57 Wade, Nicholas. "Yes, red wine holds answer. Check dosage." *The New York Times.* Nov. 2, 2006. http://www.nytimes.com/2006/11/02/science/02drug.html (Accessed Aug. 24, 2008.)

58 Seligman, 2007.

59 Wade, 2006.

60 Hobbs, Christopher. *Foundations of Health: Healing with Herbs & Foods.* Capitola, CA: Botanica Press, 1994, p. 266

61 Wren R.C. *Potter's New Cyclopedia of Botanical Drugs & Preparations.* Essex, England: The C.W. Daniel Company Limited, 1994, p. 127.

62 The George Mateljan Foundation.

63 The George Mateljan Foundation.

64 Chaiyakunapruk N, et al. The efficacy of ginger for the prevention of postoperative nausea and vomiting: a meta-analysis. *Evid Based Nurs.* 2006

Jul;9(3):80.

65 The George Mateljan Foundation. "Ginger." *The World's Healthiest Foods.* http://www.whfoods.org/genpage.php?tname=foodspice&dbid=72#summary (Accessed Aug. 25, 2008)

66 Grzanna R, Lindmark L, Frodoza CG. Ginger--an herbal medicinal product with broad anti-inflammatory actions. *J Med Food.* 2005 Summer;8:125-32.

67 Murakami A, et al. Supression of dextran sodium sulfate-induced colitis in mice by zerumbone, a subtropical ginger sesquiterpene, and nimesulid: separately and in combination. *Biochem Pharmacol.* 2003 Oct 1;66(7):1253-61.

68 El-Abhar HS, Hammad LN, Gawad HS. Modulating effect of ginger extract on rats with ulcerative colitis. *J Ethnopharmacol.* 2008 Aug 13;118(3):367-72.

69 MedicineNet.com. "Sulfasalazine." Last editorial review: Dec. 31, 1997. http://www.medicinenet.com/sulfasalazine/article.htm (Accessed Aug. 25, 2008)

70 Krinsky NI, et al. Biologic mechanisms of the protective role of lutein and zeaxanthin in the eye. *Annu Rev Nutr.* 2003;23:171-201.

71 Tan JSL, et al. Dietary antioxidants and the long-term incidence of age-related macular degeneration: The Blue Mountains Eye Study. *Ophthalmology.* 2008 Feb;115(2):334-341.

72 Richer S, et al. Double-masked, placebo-controlled, randomized trial of lutein and antioxidant supplementation in the intervention of atrophic age-related macular degeneration: the Veterans LAST study (Lutein Antioxidant Supplementation Trial). *Optometry.* 2004 Apr;75(4):216-30.

73 Semba RD, Dagnelie G. Are lutein and zeaxanthin conditionally essential nutrients for eye health? *Med Hypotheses.* 2003 Oct;61(4):465-72.

74 Bernstein PS, et al. Resonance Raman measurement of macular carotenoids in normal subjects and in age-related macular degeneration patients. *Ophthalmology.* 2002 Oct;109(10):1780-7.

75 Schatzman, Daniel. "AREDS II Trial Under Way." *Nutritional Outlook.* http://www.nutritionaloutlook.com/article.php?ArticleID=2106 (Accessed Aug. 26, 2008)

76 NUTRAingredients.com. "Lutein research gains ground." *NUTRAingredients.com.* Nov. 20, 2002. http://www.nutraingredients.com/Research/Lutein-research-gains-ground (Accessed Aug. 26, 2008)

77 Naidu PS, Singh A, Kulkarni SK. Effect of Withania somnifera root extract on resperine-induced orofacial dyskinesia and cognitive dysfunction. *Phytother Res.* 2006 Feb;20(2):140-6.

78 Kuboyama T, Tohda C, Komatsu K. Neuritic regeneration and syn-

aptic reconstruction induced by withanolide A. *Br J Pharmacol.* 2005 Apr;144(7):961-71.

79 Tohda C. Overcoming several neurodegenerative diseases by traditional medicines: the development of therapeutic medicines and unraveling pathophysiological mechanisms. *Yakugaku Zasshi.* 2008 Aug;128(8):1159-67.

80 Parihar MS, et al. Susceptibility of hippocampus and cerebral cortex to oxidative damage in streptozotocin treated mice: prevention by extracts of Withania somnifera and Aloe vera. *J Clin Neurosci.* 2004 May;11(4):397-402.

81 Tohda C, Kuboyama T, Komatsu K. Search for natural products related to regeneration of the neuronal network. *Neurosignals.* 2005;14(1-2):34-35.

82 Kuboyama T, et al. Axon- or dendrite-predominant outgrowth induced by constituents from Ashwaganda. *Neuroreport.* 2002 Oct 7;13(14):1715-20.

83 Tohda C, Kuboyama T, Komatsu K. Dendrite extension by methanol extract of Ashwaganda (roots of Withania somnifera) in SK-N-SH cells. *Neuroreport.* 2000 Jun 26;11(9):1981-5.

84 Kuboyama T, Tohda C, Komatsu K, 2005.

85 Tohda C. 2008.

86 Kuboyama T, Tohda C, Komatsu K, 2005.

87 Kuboyama T, Tohda C, Komatsu K. Withanoside IV and its active metabolite, sominone, attenuate Abeta(25-35)-induced neurodegeneration. *Eur J Neurosci.* 2006 Mar;23(6):1417-26.

88 Schliebs R, et al. Systemic administration of defined extracts from Withania somnifera (Indian ginseng) and shilajit differentially affects cholinergic but not glutamatergic and GABAergic markers in rat brain. *Neurochem Int.* 1997 Feb;30(2):181-90.

89 Choudhary MI, et al. Withanolides, a new class of natural cholinesterase inhibitors with calcium antagonistic properties. *Biochem Biophys Res Commun.* 2005 Aug 19;334(1):276-87.

90 Vinutha B, et al. Screening of selected Indian medicinal plants for acetylcholinesterase inhibitory activity. *J Ethnopharmacol.* 2007 Jan 19;109(2):359-63.

91 Naidu PS, Singh A, Kulkarni SK. Effect of Withania somnifera root extract on resperine-induced orofacial dyskinesia and cognitive dysfunction. *Phytother Res.* 2006 Feb;20(2):140-6.

92 Parihar MS, 2004.

93 Dhuley JN. Nootropic-like effect of ashwaganda (Withania somnifera L.) in mice. *Phytother Res.* 2001 Sep;15(6):524-8.

94 Segal, Marian. "Tea: A story of serendipity." *FDA Consumer magazine.* March 1996. http://www.fda.gov/FDAC/features/296_tea.html (Accessed Aug. 27, 2008)

95 Reed, Donald J. "Antioxidants help prevent age-related loss of energy."

The Linus Pauling Institute. May, 1997. http://lpi.oregonstate.edu/sp-su97/anti.html (Accessed Aug. 27, 2008)

96 NUTRAingredients.com. "Green tea is anti-inflammatory agent." NUTRAingredients.com. Jan. 30, 2002. http://www.nutraingredients.com/Research/Green-tea-is-anti-inflammatory-agent (Accessed Aug. 27, 2008)

97 Xu J, et al. Green tea extract and its major component epigallocatechin gallate inhibits hepatitis B virus in vitro. *Antiviral Res*. 2008 Jun;78(3):242-9.

98 Song JM, Lee KH, Seong BL. Antiviral effects of catechins in green tea on influenza virus. *Antiviral Res*. 2005 Nov;68(2):66-74.

99 Cheng HY, Lin CC, Lin TC. Antiviral properties of prodelphinidin B-2 3'-O-gallate from green tea leaf. *Antivir Chem Chemother*. 2002 Jul;13(4):223-9.

100 Fassina G, et al. Polyphenolic antioxidant (-)-epigallocatechin-3-gallate from green tea as a candidate anti-HIV agent. *AIDS*. 2002 Apr 12;16(6):939-41.

101 American Academy Of Allergy, Asthma & Immunology. "Elements of green tea prevent HIV from binding to human T cells." *ScienceDaily* Nov. 14, 2003. http://www.sciencedaily.com /releases/2003/11/031113065933.htm (Accessed Aug. 27, 2008)

102 Weber JM, et al. Inhibition of adenovirus infection and adenain by green tea catechins. *Antiviral Res*. 2003 Apr;58(2):167-73.

103 Mukoyama A, et al. Inhibition of rotavirus and enterovirus infections by tea extracts. *Jpn J Med Sci Biol*. 1991 Aug;44(4):181-6.

104 Chang LK, et al. Inhibition of Epstein-Barr virus lytic cycle by (-)-epigallocatechin gallate. *Biochem Biophys Res Commun*. 2003 Feb 21;301(4):1062-8.

105 Si W, et al. Bioassay-guided purification and identification of antimicrobial components in Chinese green tea extract. *J Chromatogr A*. 2006 Sep 1;1125(2):204-10.

106 Rasheed A, Haider M. Antibacterial activity of Camellia sinensis extracts against dental caries. *Arch Pharm Res*. 1998 Jun;21(3):348-52.

107 Takabayashi F, et al. Inhibitory effect of green tea catechins in combination with sucralfate on Helicobacter pylori infection in Mongolian gerbils. *J Gastroenterol*. 2004 Jan;39(1):61-3.

108 Bombardier C, et al. Comparison of upper gastrointestinal toxicity of rofecoxib and naproxen in patients with rheumatoid arthritis. VIGOR Study Group. *N Engl J Med*. 2001 May 3;344(18):1398.

109 Siegfried, 2005.

110 Kaptchuk Ted J. *The Web That Has No Weaver*. Congdon & Weed Inc.: Chicago, 1983, p. 4.

111 Wang Z, et al. Synergistic effects of multiple natural products in pancre-

atic cancer cells. *Life Sci.* 2008 Aug 15;83(7-8):293-300.

112 Shoba G, et al. Influence of piperine on the pharmacokinetics of curcumin in animals and human volunteers. *Planta Med.* 1998;64(4):353-356.

113 de Santi C, et al. Glucuronidation of resveratrol, a natural product present in grape and wine, in the human liver. *Xenobiotica.* 2000 Nov;30(11):1047-54.

114 de Santi C, et al. Sulphation of resveratrol, a natural compound present in wine, and its inhibition by natural flavonoids. *Xenobiotica.* 2000 Sep;30(9):857-66.

115 de Santi C, et al. Sulphation of resveratrol, a natural compound present in wine, in the human liver and duodenum. *Xenobiotica.* 2000 Jun;30(6):609-17.

116 Graedon Joe, Graedon Teresa. "Guggul." People's Pharmacy. Sept. 2, 2002. http://www.healthcentral.com/peoplespharmacy/408/20645.html (Accessed Sept. 11, 2008.)

117 Graedon Joe, Graedon Teresa, 2002.

118 The George Mateljan Foundation. "Garlic." The World's Healthiest Foods. http://www.whfoods.org/genpage.php?tname=foodspice&dbid=60#he althbenefits (Accessed Sept. 11, 2008.)

119 Schliebs R, et al. Systemic administration of defined extracts from Withania somnifera (Indian Ginseng) and Shilajit differentially affects cholinergic but not glutamatergic and GABAergic markers in rat brain. *Neurochem Int.* 1997 Feb;30(2):181-90.

120 Kontush K, Schekatolina S. Vitamin E in neurodegenerative disorders: Alzheimer's disease. *Ann N Y Acad Sci.* 2004;1031:249-262.

121 Hobbs, Christopher. *Foundations of Health: Healing with Herbs & Foods.* Botanica Press: Capitola CA, 1994, p. 274.

122 Foster, Steven. "Milk thistle - Silybum marianum." *Steven Foster Group, Inc.* http://www.stevenfoster.com/education/monograph/milkthistle.html (Accessed Sept. 12, 2008.)

123 Gupta SK, et al. Lycopene attenuates oxidative stress induced experimental cataract development: an in vitro and in vivo study. *Nutrition.* 2003 Sep;19(9):794-9.

124 Alternative Medicine Review. Vaccinium myrtillus - Bilberry - Monograph: Therapeutic uses in natural medicine. *Alternative Medicine Review.* Oct, 2001.

125 Lieberman Shari, Bruning Nancy. *The Real Vitamin & Mineral Book.* The Penguin Group: New York, 2007, p. 88.

126 Weil, Andrew. *Health and Healing.* Houghton Mifflin Company: New York, 1998, p. ix.

127 Adjuvant nutrition for cancer patients. *U.S. Research Reports.* Jan. 15, 1993.

128 NUTRAingredients.com. "Green tea shows superbug-battling potential."

NUTRAingredients.com. April 1, 2008 http://www.nutraingredients.com/Research/Green-tea-shows-superbug-battling-potential (Accessed Sept. 17, 2008.)

129 Knoops KTB. Mediterranean diet, lifestyle factors, and 10-year mortality in elderly European men and women. *JAMA*. 2004;292(12):1433-1439.

130 Futterman LG. Regular physical exercise reduces cardiovascular risk. *Amer J Clin Care*. 2006;15:99-102.

131 Kasapis C, Thompson P. The effects of physical activity on serum C-reactive protein and inflammatory markers. J *Am Coll Cardiol*. 2005;45:1563-1569.

132 Wannamethee SG, et al. Physical activity and hemostatic and inflammatory variables in elderly men. *Circulation*. 2002;105:1785.

133 Reuters Health. "Even a little exercise has health benefits: study." *Reuters.com*. http://www.reuters.com/article/healthNews/idUSFLE26799320070 822?feedType=RSS&feedName=healthNews (Accessed Sept. 7, 2008.)

134 Stein Rob. "Scientists finding out what losing sleep does to a body." *The Washington Post*. Oct. 9, 2005. http://www.washingtonpost.com/wp-dyn/content/article/2005/10/08/AR2005100801405.html (Accessed Sept. 7, 2008.)

135 Irwin MR, et al. Sleep deprivation and activation of morning levels of cellular and genomic markers of inflammation. *Arch Intern Med*. 2006 Sep 18:166(16):1756-62.

136 U.S. Environmental Protection Agency. "Organic gases (Volatile organic compounds - VOCs)." *U.S. Environmental Protection Agency, Indoor Air Quality*. Last updated Nov. 14, 2007. http://www.epa.gov/iaq/voc.html (Accessed Sept. 7, 2008.)

137 Lyman, Francesca. "Our bodies, our landfills?" *MSNBC*. Nov. 4, 2003. http://www.msnbc.msn.com/id/3076636/ (Accessed Sept. 10, 2008.)

138 Wegman Keith. "Can you completely relax with environmental toxins in your body?" *Edge Life magazine*. July 2006. http://www.maharishi.co.uk/selfcare/AyurvedaPanchakarmaAndEliminatingEnvironmentalToxins.htm (Accessed Sept. 9, 2008.)

139 Britt, Robert Roy. "Study: Optimists live longer." *Live Science*. Nov. 1, 2004. http://www.livescience.com/health/041101_optimist_heart.html (Accessed Sept. 7, 2008.)

140 Meggs, p. 159.

141 Lemley Brad." Shiny happy people." *Discover*. Aug. 1, 2006. http://discovermagazine.com/2006/aug/shinyhappy/article_view?b_start:int=1&-C= (Accessed Sept. 7, 2008.)

142 Seligman, Martin. *Authentic Happiness: Using the New Positive Psychology to Realize Your Potential for Lasting Fulfillment*. The Free Press: New York, 2002, p. 168.

Other Books by Safe Goods

The ADD and ADHD Diet Expanded	$ 10.95 US
ADD, The Natural Approach	$ 5.95 US
Testosterone is your Friend	$ 8.95 US
Eye Care Naturally	$ 8.95 US
The Natural Prostate Cure	$ 6.95 US
Create a Miracle with hexagonal water	$ 9.95 US
The Smart Brain Train	$ 7.95 US
New Hope for Serious Diseases	$ 7.95 US
What is Beta Glucan?	$ 4.95 US
Cancer Disarmed Expanded	$ 7.95 US
The Vertical System	$ 9.95 US
Overcoming Senior Moments Expanded	$ 9.95 US
Crissy the CowPot Gets Her Wish!	$ 9.95 US
Lower Cholesterol without Drugs	$ 6.95 US
The Secrets of Staying Young	$ 11.95 US
Worse Than Global Warming	$ 9.95 US
2012 Airborne Prophesy	$ 16.95 US
The Natural Diabetes Cure	$ 8.95 US
Rx for Computer Eyes	$ 8.95 US
Kids First: Health with No Interference	$ 16.95 US

For a complete listing of books visit our web site:
www.safegoodspub.com to order or call (888) 628-8731
for a free catalog (888) NATURE-1

NOTES

NOTES

NOTES

NOTES